Transformational Weight Loss

A personal revolution for food and body sanity

Charles Eisenstein

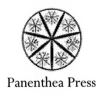

Panenthea Press

Every need brings in what's needed.
Pain bears its cure like a child.

-- Rumi

Table of Contents

Chapter One

Introduction

This book is primarily for overweight and obese people, in particular those who cannot seem to control their eating. If you are fat and find it impossible to control the amount you eat or the foods you choose, then this book is for you. It is also for anyone who cannot seem to stay on a program of exercise. It is especially for you if you are in a state of desperation or despair, if you have tried everything under the sun to lose weight and, in the long run, failed every time.

I say "the long run" because every fat person I know has had partial, temporary success at least once. That's why all the diet books out there are so popular. They work—temporarily. You can lose 40, 80, even 120 pounds on a diet of control and restriction. The problem is that when you run into a rough spot in your life, you lose control and put all the weight back on, and then some. That's what is missing from those before and after photos. What about the "after the after" photo?

This book will explain the fatal flaw in diets based on control or restriction. And it will offer an alternative that is easy, natural, and that resonates deeply with your common sense. I have a very ambitious goal in writing this book: to transform your eating habits, your body, and your life dramatically and permanently. I am not going to tell you what to eat and what not to eat. This book goes deeper than that. Instead I will show you how to realize for yourself what foods truly nourish your body, and to choose them effortlessly, without self-discipline or willpower. This book will be fundamentally different from anything you have ever tried before.

You have probably been told that your problem is that you lack motivation and self-control; that you are lazy or indulgent or weak-willed or ignorant, and that's why you are fat. You have been told it in a thousand ways, by a thousand judgmental glances as you push your cart through the supermarket, even when you walk into a room. Reading this book, you will see how it is not true. You already know it in your heart. You know that you have done your best. Soon you will bring this knowledge into your life.

The same goes for exercise as for food. This book is also for people who have ultimately failed to maintain every exercise program they've tried. I will show you how to free yourself forever from the drudgery of burning calories, and unlock the natural joy of movement.

It may surprise you to know that some obese people actually eat very little. Is this information comforting to you or alarming? It might be both, because it means that the key to healing your condition is bigger than changing what you eat or how you eat. The change will go deeper than that. You will not find a magic formula that allows you to change your diet and leaves the rest of your life the same. A saying goes, "You cannot change one thing without changing everything." The result of this book will be a life, a body, and a relationship to food so different from what you have known, that you may hardly recognize yourself.

This book is especially for the obese, but anyone who struggles with food, exercise, or health may gain some valuable insights. Anyone who suffers from poor health due to uncontrollable urges to eat too much food or the wrong food will benefit from this book. If you are at a point of confusion or despair, so much the better.

Chapter Two

Freedom from Motivation

Let's start with some good news and some bad news. The good news and the bad news is one and the same. It is that the solution I will offer you is not going to be to control your eating habits. Why is that bad news? Because trying to control your eating is safe and familiar territory. It is something you have certainly tried before. In fact you've probably tried it many, many times. Maybe you even try it every day. Maybe you were expecting this to be a motivational book that would inspire you to try even harder this time.

No. This is not a motivational book. That is good news, precisely because you've already been motivated, motivated to try again and again. You've tried, and it hasn't worked. How many years have you tried one motivational technique after another, only to fail in the long run? Oh, you've tried all right. In fact you've tried very, very hard. Thin people might look at your plate or your shopping cart or your body, and assume that you must be lazy, weak, greedy, undisciplined, or simply just not trying. People often assume that about you—hey, maybe you even assume that about yourself. It is this assumption that prompts people to offer motivation after motivation. They will tell you various tricks to control your appetite. They might try "tough love", the boot camp approach, hoping that your own self-disgust will motivate you to try harder.

It is easy to understand how the logic of trying harder gets started. Trying hard actually does work—for a while. You lose 20, 40 pounds and you feel great. You feel good in your body and you feel good about yourself. You derive self-esteem from your success. But eventually, the cravings and appetites you have tried so hard to suppress come back with a vengeance. It can happen at any moment of weakness. Often it happens when there is some kind of upheaval in your life, perhaps when you lose your job, or when you have relationship troubles, or when you have a health problem. In the face of a personal crisis, the effort of control can just become too much to handle. Your weight balloons back up to what it was before, with a few extra pounds for good measure.

At this point, you naturally conclude, "It happened because I stopped trying," or, "It happened because I didn't try hard enough." Eventually you decide to try again—harder this time—and you experience the same result: failure. You conclude, therefore, that you just must be weak. This pattern confirms your supposed weakness again and again.

This leads to the first key insight of Transformational Weight Loss. It is a different way to interpret the yo-yo diet pattern of repeated failure. Before you decide to go another round, consider this: If trying hard didn't work, then isn't trying harder doing more of what doesn't work? It is like the man who tried to run to the horizon. The faster he ran, the faster it receded, so he concluded he just wasn't running fast enough. Eventually, after a lifetime of running, he found himself back at his starting point.

Lets face it: control doesn't work. If it worked, you would have a different body than the one you have today. Control doesn't work, it never has worked, and it isn't going to work. This would be terrible news if there weren't another way. That is what I will offer you in this book, a way to transform your body and your life that does not depend on willpower, control, or trying harder.

I want you to know that at least one thin person (me) knows your countless struggles, knows how very hard you have tried, and doesn't see you as weak, lazy, greedy, or self-indulgent. The reason I don't see you that way is that I *know* you are not that way—even if you think you are. I know it beyond a shadow of a doubt, and you will realize it as well when you understand the alternative explanation I will offer.

By the way, not only do I know that you are not lazy and weak, I think you are heroic. I think that for two reasons. One is your indomitable spirit. Through all those years, no matter how beaten down you were, no matter how discouraged, you still found the strength to try and try again. You refused to believe that it had to be this way. You heroically refused to settle for obesity. In the midst of despair, you even learned to find joy and hope. Very few thin people know the incredible strength of spirit you have built through these struggles. Very few thin people know what it is like to be in a society where most people judge you, degrade you, and even insult you on a daily basis.

The second reason I think you are heroic is that you have taken on a huge and difficult challenge. Only a very powerful, noble, courageous soul would choose to be born into the circumstances you have chosen and the body that you have been. Of course, you may not be aware of having made this choice, but on a deep unconscious level you chose these circumstances because you were ready to take them on. You were ready for the spiritual growth that is available through experiencing and transcending the conditions of your life.

Many of you reading this book are ready to move on now from that state of being. You are ready to no longer be obese. You are ready because you have fully experienced and integrated the condition of obesity. Did you know that an essential part of that experience is the despair and hopelessness and hell of it? Without that, your experience would not be complete. Now I sense that many of you are nearing the point of complete surrender. That is when you despair of yet another bout of trying hard, and you just *give up*. You simply don't know any more. You reach a state of emptiness. This state of emptiness is what will invite in something new. Unless you are close to that state, you probably won't resonate with the message of this book. That is okay with me. I truly do not want you to follow my suggestions unless they feel right to you.

The state of surrender I just mentioned is not the same as "accepting that this is just the way I am." Yes, self-acceptance is a big part of what I will offer you, but part of that is also accepting that the self can change. The surrender is not a surrender to being like this forever. It is actually a bigger surrender than that. It is more like, "I know life can be different and I can be healthy, I know it is possible but I just don't know how to get there and I'm sick and tired of trying."

Your situation is like the man locked in a room with no roof. He has felt along the walls, seeking an exit, seeking a weak point, digging and scraping with all his might for a very

long time. Finally he gives up. Still believing deep down there
is a way out, but having completely exhausted every possibility, he sits down in despair and raises his head. The walls are
only six feet high. The exit was available the whole time. All
he had to do is look up.

In a sense, your situation is hopeless. Your experience
has already proven that, proven that no amount of trying will
make and keep you thin. So are you ready for something else?
Are you ready to look up? Are you ready to enter a new way
of living and being? Because a change is possible in your near
future that is so profound that life as you have known it will
seem like a bad dream that fades rapidly upon waking. Your
body and your experience of being alive can change so much
that you might feel like you have been reborn in a different
body. Indeed, something will have died and something will
have been born, because you will be entering new and unfa-
miliar territory. The death of the familiar, a birth into something new—that is something that's always a little bit scary.
When you read what I am about to share with you, you might
feel a strong fear response. The core of this work is so auda-
cious that it is truly scary. But at the same time, you should
feel a sense of boldness too, boldness and exhilaration. If you
do not, then please respect your fear and wait until you are
ready.

Fear has a bad reputation in spiritual circles. Often it is
described as the opposite of love. But fear has its purpose
too. We create for ourselves a cocoon or a womb of our
fears, a safe space in which we can grow. Eventually we grow
to the limits of that space, and the fears that once protected
us become confining. Eventually we can no longer stand the
smallness of the familiar space we inhabited, and we are born

into something new. If you are ready for this work, the kind of fear you will feel is like that of a young child, about to enter the water for the first time. She really wants to go in, she is ready, yet she is afraid. If the fear you feel is more akin to the child being taunted by teenagers to take a high dive off the rocks, knowing she shouldn't but afraid to say no, then please respect that feeling. File this information away, mull it over, and perhaps someday you will feel the true desire to take the plunge.

Chapter Three

The Great Release

Because control hasn't worked, I'm going to invite you to release control. Because the struggle against your self hasn't worked, I'm going to invite you to cease the struggle. Because you have tried and tried without lasting success, I'm going to invite you to stop trying. I'm just being realistic here. Control hasn't worked! Insanity has been defined as doing the same thing again and again while hoping for different results. Let's not continue the madness. I am going to offer you an alternative. You can call it self-trust.

Self-trust means to love and trust your body unconditionally. More specifically, it means to love your body and to trust its messages. And what are the body's messages? We call them feelings. It is how it feels to be you at a given time. For the purposes of this book, the relevant feelings are things like pleasure, desire, deliciousness, revulsion, discomfort, satisfaction, and delight. But really it comes down to the first two: pleasure and desire.

I would like to identify a voice of fear and self-*distrust* that may be speaking to you right now. It says, "Wait a minute! I can't let go of control and struggle. After all, every time I lose control, look what happens! I eat a whole box of cookies. A whole bag of chips. An enormous quantity of food. It's only that tiny amount of self-control I *do* have that stops me from ballooning to double what I am now."

This fear seems perfectly logical, but actually it is built upon an illusion. What you are seeing is the result of losing control, not the result of living without control. When you deny true desire for a long time, the pressure builds and builds until eventually it explodes out uncontrollably. Another way of putting it is that in the war against the self, you lose every time.

In the next chapter I will explain why it *seems* that the body and its desires and pleasures lead us astray. I will explain why it *seems* that desire unleashed causes you to eat too much food or the wrong food.

Self-control reminds me of the man with a leaky pressure cooker. The little hole where the steam is supposed to escape was blocked, so the steam kept escaping from little cracks in the seal. Each time this happened, the man welded the crack shut. As the pressure rose, new leaks kept springing open, and the man welded them shut again. He welded a whole new layer of metal onto the pressure cooker in a desperate attempt to prevent the steam from ever escaping. Well, you can imagine what happened in the end.

The steam in this story represents desire. This book will teach you how to open the proper pathway for desire to flow through. It is not about the conquest of desire. That would not be self-trust, that would be a continuation of the war against the self. Besides, it doesn't work, remember? Eventually you "explode" into uncontrollable bingeing.

The other part of self-trust—to unconditionally love and accept yourself—has almost become a cliché these days. Everyone at least pays lip service to unconditional self-acceptance. However, I have met very few people who enact it to any meaningful degree. Later in this book I will offer some tools to reveal and heal the hidden ways in which we reject and deny ourselves literally a thousand times a day. For now, though, just consider: Do you love yourself? All of yourself? Do you love and accept your body? Your fat? Your appearance?

If you notice any self-disgust or any other kind of self-hatred, including self-hating beliefs in your own laziness, greediness, or weakness, then I have a very big request of you. I request that you love and accept your self-hatred too. I want you to accept not just your body, but all of your habits, thoughts, and feelings as the perfectly natural response to the life you chose to enter.

Got that? Self-hatred and self-rejection are not the new enemy, to be hated or rejected. You will not transcend these beliefs, nor will you transform your body, by fighting and rejecting them. Instead, be okay with where you are right now. This is the starting point. Be okay with where you are, be okay with who you are, and be ready to say goodbye to that. Because you are about to enter a very different state of being.

Chapter Four

Substitute Desires

Now it is time to answer the riddle, "Why does it seem that the body and its desires lead us astray? What does it seem that the things we want end up hurting ourselves and others?"

This entire book hinges on answering this riddle in a satisfactory way. If desire is the enemy, then self-trust is foolish. If desire is the enemy, you must always be on guard against yourself. And since desires come from the body, the body becomes an enemy too, and the war against the self is perfectly rational.

The reason that your desire for food appears to be a problem is that you are using food as a substitute for what you really want and need. The true need could be an emotional or spiritual need, or it could be a nutritional need that your current diet cannot meet. We'll discuss nutrition later in the book, but I want to explore non-nutritional needs first, because for many people they are more important. For many people, correct nutritional knowledge simply does not help. They will follow a great diet all day and eat an entire box of cookies as they relax in the evening. They will follow a great diet all week and then eat all the food in the house.

What are the needs for which food substitutes? I think the most important ones are love, intimacy, excitement, connection, self-expression, adventure, identity, and security. The following diagram shows how the desire for all of these things gets diverted onto food.

Figure 1: Substitute Desires

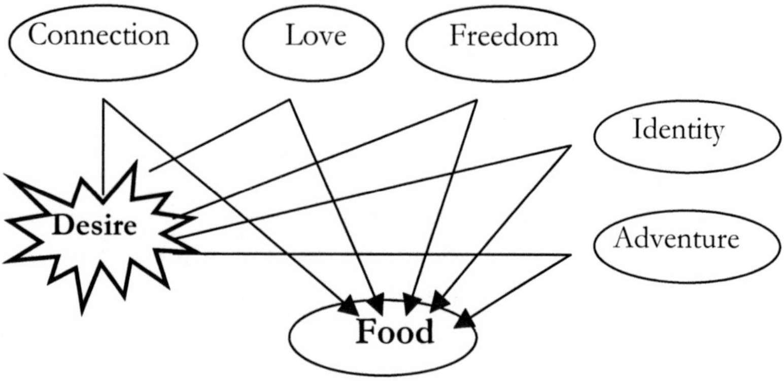

Access to the true needs is blocked, so the desire is deflected onto food.

Let's start with the example of the sweet and sugary foods that are one of the main objects of bingeing and food cravings. The urge to overindulge in sweet snacks is utterly overpowering for many people, even when they know that sugar is harming their bodies. I don't think most people are actually as ignorant as nutritional educators tend to assume. People know sugar is bad for them, but the prospect of doing without is so daunting that they prefer not to think about it too much. They'd rather not go there.

The reason that sugar is so addictive is that people use it as a substitute for something they really need. Very often, that something is love. Living in this lonely society, with its broken families and shattered communities, its hyper-competitiveness and its depersonalization, many of us are actually starving for love. We don't get nearly the amount of love and affection that we need. Now, it has been said that love is the sweetest thing in the world. That's why we call our lovers "sweetheart" and our babies "sweetie-pie". So if we are starving for love, we are also starving for sweetness. The love is unavailable, so instead we turn to the nearest substitute for love's sweetness. You know what that is—sugar!

The use of sugar to substitute for love often starts in childhood, when our parents give us sweet treats as rewards for good behavior or as their way of showing love. Many of us suffer a damaged capacity to fully express love. Moreover, the stresses of modern life often make parents too busy to show love through quality time with their children. To make matters worse, when we are busy and stressed, we might be more likely to ignore or shout at our children. Because of all of this, many parents use treats to show love. You yell at Junior and make him cry, so you give him a lollipop to make up for it. Your parents wanted to give you love, they wanted to be good to you, and maybe just about the only way they knew how, or the only way they had time for, was to give you a cookie. And so, early on, you may have come to associate sugar with love.

By adulthood, this habit may be deeply ingrained. Sugar = Love. With your true need for love unfulfilled, naturally you give yourself the sweets. Think about the connotations of the word "treat" and the word "dessert". A treat is something you get for being good. It is something you get because you are special. A special treat, just for you. It is a primal way of being good to yourself. As for a dessert, the word actually means "something you deserve." Why do you deserve it? You deserve it because you are good. Maybe you deserve it because you stayed on your diet all day. Maybe you deserve it because you had a hard day. Maybe you deserve it because you lost your job. Maybe you deserve it because your boyfriend left you. Maybe you deserve it because it is Friday and you deserve to celebrate.

These examples point to an even deeper level of the need to receive love. In fact, we are not dependent on the outside world to meet the need for love. The true need is for self-love. That is really what we are trying to do when we give ourselves a treat or a dessert. Or ten treats or ten desserts. That might be the only vehicle we have to show ourselves love. Other people might use other vehicles, such as smoking or drugs or shopping, and they will perhaps not be obese, but they will surely have other problems in their lives.

Your inner self, your inner child has such a powerful need to receive love that the desires it generates are unstoppable. No amount of willpower can thwart them. So suppose you go on a diet and decide to cut out all sugar. Well, the need for love, that you had been indirectly meeting with sugar, is now unmet. An unmet need generates desire, and the longer the need is not met, the stronger the desire grows. It is just like the pressure cooker. Finally, perhaps in a moment of weakness, the desire explodes outward and you empty the entire cupboard.

Desires come from unmet needs. If you hold your breath, you will soon feel a strong desire to breathe. That desire comes from your body's need for oxygen. If you do not drink water, you will soon feel a strong desire to drink. If you are starving, you will have a strong desire to eat. Unmet needs generate desires.

It is the same with love. It is one of the most powerful needs there is. If you had been using sugar to meet that need, and then you cut out the sugar, your desire will grow and grow until it becomes uncontrollable—unless you find another way to meet the need. That is why addicts sometimes quit one drug only to replace it with another. A much better outcome is to meet the true need directly. In this case, the true need wasn't for sugar, it was for love. If you can meet that need, then the craving for sugar can disappear like magic. It just isn't there any more, and the only discipline you need is a very gentle mindfulness so as not to eat it out of habit.

If you think back on your dieting history, you might find that periods of success actually coincide with other things that were working in your life. Maybe you were in an exciting phase of a new job or relationship. Maybe something else was fulfilling the needs that you'd been using food to substitute for.

As you can see, desire is not the real culprit here. The culprit, the fuel for the cravings, is actually desire denied, desire contorted, and desire displaced onto something that can never meet the real need. No matter how much sugar you eat, you aren't actually receiving the love you need. Therefore, sugar is addictive. Anything is addictive if it appears to meet a need, but actually numbs the pain from that need while leaving it unmet.

An unmet need hurts. When its needs are not met, an organism experiences distress. In fact that is the biological origin and purpose of pain—to guide us away from activities and behavior that are harmful, for example touching a hot candle flame or holding your breath for a long time. We will return to this theme in a later chapter.

Figure 2: Unmet Needs – normal pattern

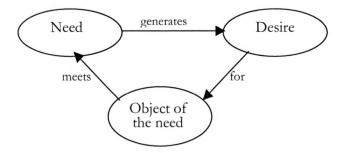

Be at peace with your desires. They come from a valid source.

Figure 3: Unmet Needs – addiction pattern

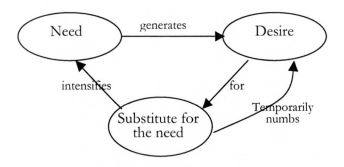

Another need for which food substitutes is the need for self-expression. When we are in a vocation or a relationship where this need is not met, we experience considerable distress, a constant low-level anxiety or discomfort. Imagine yourself sitting in front of a computer inputting data, data that you have no personal interest in. Perhaps you have been hired to input data on a company's customers. Hour after hour, entry after entry—the boredom is excruciating. You have no desire to do this; deep down a voice is saying, "I was not put here on earth to input data." And now imagine a bag of chips right next to the computer. If you are like most people, you will constantly reach for the chips to momentarily escape the tedium of your job.

So again, it is not that you have a true desire for chips, and that your body's desire is betraying you by wanting the wrong foods. No, your desire is actually for distraction, for an escape. Digging another level deeper, your desire is to be doing something that engages your creativity and intellect. You don't have that, so you reach for the nearest substitute. Potato chips. At least they take you away from what you don't want to be doing.

More generally, we can use food as a temporary escape from a situation that is not in alignment with our true being. This is actually one of the major causes of overeating. You don't want to stop eating, you don't want to get up from the table because that means you are going back to a life that on some level you do not want to live. Anything to delay that! Anything to delay going back to life. Another helping, a dessert. This kind of eating pattern is common in unhappy marriages, and it often afflicts both partners. As long as you are standing in the buffet line, all is well. As long as there is a bag of Snickers Bars on hand, all is well. All that you need do whenever the discomfort of unmet relationship needs arises is to pop something in your mouth. So again, here is a deep unmet need coming out as a desire for food. But that is not the true desire.

A related unmet need that often generates eating problems is the need for excitement. For some people, mealtime is the high point of their day. This is not because they love food too much. It is because they are stuck in a life that is fundamentally unexciting to them. It is quite understandable. The dreams and ambitions and big plans of adolescence fade into the monotony and routine of adulthood. We fall into boring jobs and take comfort in predictable routines. We put a high value on security and stop taking risks in life. But a human being needs adventure. We need to explore our world, expand our boundaries, and experience novelty. If this need is not met, once again we might use food as a substitute. A poor substitute, but a substitute nonetheless.

You can tell that you are using food as a substitute for excitement if you notice yourself constantly looking forward to your next meal or snack. Sometimes, even while you are still eating a snack, your mind will have already begun thinking of the next one. You start thinking of dessert while you are still eating dinner, taking comfort in the fact that there is still one more course to go. You might start associating food with fun and excitement. It's party time!

You may have noticed that advertisers take advantage of our unmet need for excitement by associating food with images of fun and adventure. This is especially the case in T.V. commercials for snack food and fast food restaurants. Ah, here is the answer to your boredom!

Once again, no matter how much exciting food you eat, your true desire for adventure, to explore your world and expand your boundaries, is not going to be met. It will be there underneath, continuing to drive the craving for more and more exciting snacks. You can apply all the willpower you want, but it won't do any good if the true desire goes unmet.

In our society, perhaps the most pervasive unmet need is the need for connection. More than any other society that has ever existed, we are separate from nature and separate from each other. Gone are the days when we lived in small towns or villages and knew the stories of everyone around us. Gone are the days when all of our needs—for food, shelter, clothing, and entertainment—were met by people we knew personally. Today we live by and large in a world of strangers. You probably are not personally acquainted with the person who grew your food, made your clothes, built your house, sang the songs on your iPod, or formulated your medicine. Even food preparation has become the province of strangers, as some 60% of all meals are now prepared outside the home, in restaurants or supermarket delis.

We have also become separated from the world of nature. We no longer know the names, habits, and other qualities of the plants, animals, and soils that surround us. At best, nature for most of us is but a spectacle. Scenery. But we were meant to be intimately familiar with all the life around us, as well as with the land where we lived. For a primitive person or a Medieval villager, every hill, every natural scent, every local plant and animal, every insect and bird, as well as the clouds, the weather, the stars and the seasons were all intimate companions.

The loss of most of these connections leaves us with a terrible incompleteness and a crying need to reconnect. But there are few chances to do so in the artificial world of technology. For many of us, one of the only ways left to reconnect is through food.

In other words, we eat because we are lonely.

Certainly it helps mitigate the loneliness if we have a loving partner and a good family life, but often that is not enough to compensate for the loss of connection to nature and community. Loneliness is built in to modern lifestyles. When people become food-obsessed, the driving unmet need is often the need for connection. Sometimes, food is all that is available to meet that need. Food indeed puts us into intimate connection with the rest of the living universe. Unless you have learned to photosynthesize, all food originates as a living animal, plant, or fungus. When you eat, you are connecting to other life forms in a most direct, basic way.

Unfortunately, food can only satisfy a very small part of our need for connection. It cannot satisfy our need to see the stars in a darkened sky. It cannot satisfy our need to feel our feet in the mud and smell the odor of fresh soil. It cannot meet our need to be familiar with the songs of a hundred birds. It cannot meet our need to recognize by sight the diversity of life around us. It cannot meet the need for frequent touch and affection from other human beings. It cannot meet the need to care and be cared for on a physical and emotional level by those who know us well. All of these needs for connection, and many more, we transfer onto food. We eat more and more of it because we are indeed hungry. We are not actually hungry for food though. We are hungry for connection. We are hungry for something that food cannot provide. At least, food cannot provide nearly enough of it, no matter how much we eat. But it is perhaps the nearest substitute available, so we eat and eat and eat. But no matter how much we eat, we are never truly satisfied. Have you ever had that experience? Have you ever eaten until you were bursting at the gills, yet still felt unsatisfied? You still felt like you wanted more. Perhaps you concluded that you must be incredibly greedy, to be completely stuffed and still want more.

You wanted more, all right. It's just that it was not food that you wanted more of. But since food was all that was available, you kept eating. That is how we become enslaved to food.

There are other needs that we attempt to meet with food. Some people use it as a substitute for self-approval. Perhaps they internalized parental praise for eating a lot. "Be a good girl and finish your plate." Some people use food as a substitute for empowerment, autonomy, or freedom. The refrigerator becomes their playground, a domain where they are the king. (Anorexics do something similar, except they use self-denial of food as a substitute for autonomy and freedom.) If this is you, have compassion for yourself! Don't say, "I'm just going to have to stop using food to substitute for freedom." See it instead as just a symptom pointing you toward the real lack in your life. Because you are meant to be the king of your life!

Some people use food for identity. Identity—a sense of who we are—is a very basic need. It is related to the need for connection, because we know who we are through our relationships. In a lonely and alienated society, we may cling to eating patterns that tell us who we are. It might be the way we ate in our families growing up. Certain foods make us feel at home, providing a sense of security and *familiarity* (of the family). We also might associate certain foods or eating patterns with an ethnic identity such as Italian or Jewish. To leave family or cultural eating habits behind can be uncomfortable, because you are leaving behind part of yourself, part of your identity. You are becoming someone new.

Often when this happens, people will slip into a new food-based identity. They derive identity and a sense of self-worth by being a vegetarian, a raw foodist, or a follower of some other diet. I am suggesting something radically different: to let food just be food.

Trying to meet the need for love, self-expression, or excitement with food is like trying to assuage thirst by eating ice cream. While you are eating it, your throat feels cool, but afterwards you are even thirstier. So you do what worked last time—have another ice cream cone! While you are having it you feel good again, although maybe not quite as good as before. The underlying need gets stronger and stronger.

The same thing happens when we attempt to use food to meet non-food needs. It appears to work. We feel better for a moment. But after the food has been consumed, the original need is still there, perhaps even stronger than ever. The question, then, is how can we identify the true need? How can the thirsty ice cream eater discover that what she really wants is water? To answer this question, I would like to first introduce you to an utterly simple truth.

Chapter Five

Self-forcing

Here is a truth that will never change: it feels good to meet your needs. This is simply basic biology. If you hold your breath for a minute, it feels good to take a breath. If you are thirsty, it feels good to drink, and if you are hungry it feels good to eat. When you are cold, a warm fire feels good; when you are sad it feels good to be hugged, and when you are lonely, it feels good to receive an unexpected phone call from an old friend.

Can you imagine a universe where this were not true? Imagine that it didn't feel good to drink when thirsty. There you are, noticing the sensations of dehydration, and you think, "Well, I really don't want to drink, but I know I should, because if I don't my intracellular electrolyte concentration will rise, my blood will thicken... sooner or later I will die. Oh, all right, I guess I'd better drink something."

Imagine that breathing didn't feel good. You think, "Gee, it's been half a minute since I've taken a breath. My oxygen level is getting low, interfering with my neurons' ability to function. All right, all right, I guess I'd better take a breath. There. (Ten seconds later...) Now I have to do it again? What a chore. Again and again and again."

From these two (admittedly silly) examples, you can see what happens when unmet needs become disconnected from pleasure and desire—we must live by incentive and threat instead. This is not a purely hypothetical scenario. In fact, this is how most modern people live their lives. In many areas of life, we no longer do what we truly desire to do, and we think it is necessary to sacrifice pleasure to obtain future benefits.

How do we make ourselves do something we do not actually want to do? Again, it is through incentives and threats. We say, "I would like to sleep in, but if I do my boss will be angry and I might not get a raise. I might get fired. If I arrive on time I will get approval. So I'd better make myself get out of bed."

We say, "I'd really like to eat a box of cookies right now, but if I do that I will get fatter, and if I eat these celery sticks instead I'll get thinner. So I'd better not do what I want to."

The college student says, "I'd really like to go out and party now, but if I do I won't be able to study for the exam next Tuesday, and I'll get a worse grade, and my GPA will go down, and my parents will be upset, and I won't get as good a job." Reluctantly, she stays in.

All of these are what I call self-forcing. Force is what is necessary to make someone act contrary to his or her desires. The essence of self-forcing is fear.

How to you force someone to do something? At its most extreme, force means a threat to someone's life. The force we use upon ourselves to fight desire and pleasure is different in degree but not in kind. "Do it, or else."

The most common form this self-forcing takes is through self-approval and disapproval. The incentive is, "Do it and I will give myself love and approval." You stay on a diet all day, withholding from yourself all your favorite foods, and what is your reward? Your reward is that you get to approve of yourself. You get to say, "I was good today." You get to give yourself love.

And if you cheat on your diet, then you do the opposite. You feel guilty or ashamed. Guilt is essentially the feeling, "I did wrong," and shame is, "I am bad." You do not approve of yourself. You do not give yourself love. You say to yourself, "I am wrong, I am bad, I am weak, I am greedy..." You think that if you beat yourself up enough, then next time you won't dare cheat on your diet.

Is this mentality of punishment and praise familiar to you? It originates in childhood, because this is how parents, teachers, and society at large try to control the natural expression of our desires. The most frightening threat to a child (or any young mammal) is the threat of parental abandonment. When a mother withholds her love and approval, she is tapping into a child's greatest fear. More than anything else, a child wants to be accepted by her parents. That means she will try very, very hard to control herself if that is what it takes to be a "good girl."

When we grow up, we internalize the conditional approval and rejection of our parents. We can then force ourselves to act counter to our desires. We force ourselves with the threat of withholding self-love, and the incentive of allowing self-love. Instead of following a diversity of natural desires, we are governed by a single overpowering desire for self-approval, for self-love. We constantly strive to maintain an image of ourselves as right and good.

When self-love is conditional, people will do almost anything to obtain it. For generals and politicians, the need to see themselves as right may be so strong that they will send thousands to their deaths rather than admit that they were wrong. Other people (anorexics) will starve themselves to death in order to receive their daily dose of self-approval.

Another dimension of self-forcing that may be familiar to you is rebellion. You are possessed of a strong spirit that rebels against control. When the control comes from the outside, in the form of parental threats coded as approval and rejection, then children and especially teenagers will rebel against authority figures. They are not consciously aware of the reason for their rebellion. It is an unreasoning and uncontrollable "No!" When it comes to adult food issues, the same response manifests as a voice that says, "Oh yeah? I'm gonna have whatever I want! Don't tell me what to eat." You might notice a voice like this at the beginning of a binge. We are divine, autonomous beings, not meant to live a life under the control of others. The spirit protests against that. The inner regime of incentive, shame and guilt originates in external control over our selves, so of course we rebel against it. We are not meant to be slaves.

Perhaps this explanation of bingeing will help you find some self-acceptance. Bingeing is not a sign of weakness; actually it is a sign of strength. It is your unconquerable spirit throwing off its shackles. No one is going to control you; no one can. The problem is not the rebellion, it is the way the rebellion is expressed. The primal hunger of the spirit for autonomous self-expression is turned toward food. If you become clear about the true target of the rebellion, then you will no longer express it through bingeing. The true target of the rebellion is the tyranny of self-forcing. And the tyrant is the Judge, constantly evaluating whether you are good or bad, and meting out self-praise or self-criticism as a result.

It is time to fire that judge! It is time for a revolution against that tyrant! Transformational weight loss is entirely based on self-acceptance and self-trust. The constant evaluation and criticism has not worked. Goading yourself into action has not worked. Scaring yourself into eating less has not worked. Motivating yourself to diet and exercise has not worked. There may have been times when you have resigned yourself to being fat forever. That is a positive first step, but it is only a first step, because you know in your heart that vitality and health are your birthright. This is what you will ultimately accept through self-acceptance. What is this "self" that you are accepting? The self you have been, or the self that is emerging? Or both?

Chapter Six

Self-acceptance

The self-acceptance that will transform your life is very different from resigning yourself to being fat forever. Yet, it does not reject the fatness, nor does it reject any of the behaviors that led to it. It does not seek to force a change to those behaviors.

True self-acceptance is to look in the mirror and say, "My body is the perfect adaptation to everything I have experienced." Once upon a time you were a child, and you were perfect. Who knows why you grew fat? Maybe you know, or maybe you have read some theories but none ring true yet. Could it be "armoring", the adding on of layer after layer of shielding against a cold, cruel world? Could it be a fear of intimacy, borne of betrayal when you were young and vulnerable? Could it be as I have described, overeating to reassure yourself of connection in a lonely, alienated world? Could it be, very mundanely, that you are malnourished, unable to absorb nutrients and therefore eating as much food as possible in a desperate attempt to feed yourself? You may not consciously know which answer is right—maybe they all are— but rest assured that your body does know.

The condition of your body is not an error. It is the perfect response to all that you have experienced. The same thing goes for your behaviors and beliefs. The baby you was thrust into this world, and has responded as best she or he could. You came here with nothing. You were completely helpless, emotionally and physically defenseless, and there is much pain in this world. You responded as best you could. Even your self-judgment, self-criticism, and self-hatred are totally understandable. They are exactly how an innocent child learns to cope with the circumstances of our culture. For a toddler, the mother is the universe to her. What happens when the universe rejects her? The conclusion, "I am bad" is totally reasonable.

I do not mean to imply that you had particularly bad parents. They loved you and did the best they could to express and enact that love from their own damaged state. The rejection, shaming, and threat of conditional approval we exercise on children is so deeply woven into our culture that we are seldom aware of it. Do not blame yourself and do not blame your parents. Everything you did and everything you are is merely a response to what was. The same for your parents, and their parents, and the whole world. This is what I mean by self-acceptance. It is nothing less than forgiveness. You forgive yourself for what you are. By extension, you forgive everyone else for what they did.

By accepting yourself as the perfect adaptation to what *was*, you are releasing attachment to the past. Free of the past, you are free to create a future that is different from the past. So you see, self-acceptance does not resign you to staying fat—in fact it frees you to be no longer fat.

In the next part of the book I will describe how to apply self-acceptance and self-trust directly to your experience of food. In order to empower those techniques though, I strongly suggest that you cultivate an overall state of self-acceptance in your life. This is actually very easy. Are you tempted to validate self-acceptance by making it hard? No, it is easy. Let me tell you how.

The key realization is that you do not need to force love to happen. That's because love is your true state, your default condition. All that is necessary is to become aware of it. Self-acceptance is based not on trying, but on truth. You do not have to exercise any special indulgence or allowances toward yourself. You are not doing yourself any unwarranted favor by recognizing your own fundamental goodness. You are simply recognizing the truth.

Find a mirror and look at yourself for a few minutes with the intention of seeing the good and beauty within. Very likely, you will identify various flaws in your appearance. You might even find yourself extending that criticism to your behavior, thoughts, etc. You might notice a constant stream of judgments and criticism. *Do not try to stop this flow.* Instead, just take note of it. You cannot find true self-acceptance if you do not also accept your present lack of self-acceptance. That is part of you too. Take a gentle attitude toward all of yourself.

On the one hand, stay grounded in the awareness of this book, that all you are in body and mind is the innocent, normal adaptation to the circumstances of your past. On the other hand, witness all that you are. Here is my skin. Here is my neck. Here is my self-judgment. Here is my self-hatred. Here is my blame. Here is my resentment. Here is my despair. Here is my hope. Here is my negativity. Here is my story of perpetual failure. Over the years you have developed an elaborate logic surrounding all of these things, stories upon stories upon stories. Take a break from elaborating on those, and instead just observe them.

You don't have to *do* anything about it. You don't have to do anything about the negativity and you don't have to do anything about your weight. Right now, in front of the mirror, witnessing is enough. From this witnessing, tremendous changes are going to flow. They will be natural, perhaps even effortless. When we apply the same principle to eating, dramatic changes will happen there too, again without all the trying that you know doesn't work.

I was about to write, "Take some time with a mirror, or just sitting quietly, to appreciate yourself every day." But let's face it: some days you just don't feel very appreciative of yourself. That's OK. You do not have to force it. The appreciation needn't be an effort. It is just the truth. It comes from realizing the truth about yourself and your life. So really, all that is necessary is that you witness. The self-appreciation will grow. Welcome it when it comes, be glad of it, enjoy it, but don't try to force it or cling onto it. That's not necessary, and may even be counterproductive.

So instead I will say, take some time for gentle self-witnessing, with or without a mirror, every day. Throughout the day as well, and especially in situations involving food such as shopping, cooking, or eating, maintain this witness consciousness and take note of your self-criticisms, judgments, and internal threats and incentives. Again, you don't have to DO anything about them! Often we will avoid facing the truth for fear that we'll have to do something about it. That aversion is unnecessary. The truth exercises its own power. That is not to say you will take no action. You will. It's just that the action will spring from internal motivation. It will be natural, automatic even. You will want to do it. You will hardly be able to stop yourself.

The same will happen with your relationship to food. Your desire, your true unfettered desire, will return to its natural object—the foods that meet your true needs. You will simply not desire foods that harm you, and you will not desire to overeat. Health and desire will be one. Never again will you say to yourself, "I'm going to have to *do* something about my weight."

Chapter Seven

Natural Motivation

The origins of self-forcing run deep. In order to reconnect with true desire, and to reconnect with the pleasurable good feelings that guide us to meet our needs, it is necessary to release the compulsion to measure up to your own standards of good and bad. No longer will you put yourself through painful contortions and sacrifices in order to approve of and love yourself. Instead, you will be good to yourself without deserving it. You will trust pleasure and desire, because you know that both come from real needs.

Modern adult human beings are the only creatures on the planet that purposely do things that feel bad! Babies, for instance, do not go on health food diets and they do not do workouts. A baby does not lie on the floor thinking, "Gosh, I'd really like to just keep lying here doing nothing, but then I won't develop my muscles and gross motor skills, so I guess I'd better get up and start running around." No, for a baby movement comes naturally and joyfully. Babies never need to motivate themselves, they are motivation incarnate. They are energy incarnate. They are in the full flow of life force.

How can you tap into the natural motivation and flowing life-force of a two-year-old? It won't be by trying harder to conquer your natural desires. That's not what a baby does—why do you think you must do that?

Despite a total lack of self-forcing, babies love to exert every effort to overcome challenges. Just watch a toddler trying to open a cupboard door to see what is inside. We can see from watching young children the results of true desire unleashed. We see health, vitality, creativity, dynamism. We want that for ourselves too. What insanity has led us to believe that we can achieve what babies have by doing the opposite of what babies do?

Wild animals are the same. While domestic animals absorb some of our own habits and overeat, wild animals do not, despite a superabundance of food. I used to spend time watching a woodchuck who was living in my garden, which he quickly destroyed. Despite the enormous quantity of food available to him, he did not spend all his time eating, nor did he get obese. He could have, but he did not. I do not think he was restraining himself or fighting desire. In a state of nature, when we have eaten enough we no longer desire to eat more. A woodchuck doesn't think, "I would sure like to keep eating now, but I'd better stop because it is bad for me to overeat." A woodchuck is not afraid of getting fat. A woodchuck does not exercise self-restraint. Why, then, do we think we need to exercise self-restraint to enjoy the health of a wild animal or a baby?

I have already told you the answer: substitute desires. We use food to substitute for what we really want. Therefore, no matter how much we eat, we never have enough. We think the cause of overeating is unrestrained desire. Actually it is the opposite. The cause is the blocking of desire. It is the blocking of our true desires, so that they are displaced onto food.

Because it feels good to meet our needs, and because desire comes from unmet needs, our bodies can show us the way back to true desire. The way is through pleasure. But this poses another riddle. Why does it seem that pleasure in fact guides us toward harm? Why does it seem that what feels the best is to overeat, to pig out on cookies, to stay planted on the sofa instead of moving your body?

Why does it seem that the modern adult human is the one great exception to nature's design?

Biologically, pleasure originated as a system to guide an organism toward things that benefit it. Even in a bacterium, glucose receptors on the cell membrane initiate chemical processes that cause the organism to move toward a food source. Pleasure is a biological message, mediated through our nervous system, that says, "Yes, that is meeting my needs." Discomfort or pain is the opposite message. It says, "This is damaging me." That is why pain receptors innervate nearly every square millimeter of our bodies. They are there to protect us. We touch a hot stove and before our skin cells start dying in droves, the pain receptors warn us and we jerk our hand away. We overeat, and the resulting discomfort tells us to stop, or to not do it again.

Pleasure equals Yes. Pain equals No. Biologically, it doesn't get any simpler than that. What has happened to us, that we think otherwise? What has happened to modern adults to make us think that it is good to deny ourselves pleasure?

Chapter Eight

The Second-Oldest Lie

The phrase, "No pain, no gain" encapsulates a reversal of the fundamental biological equation, Pain equals No. And it sure seems true sometimes. You undergo the "pain" of a workout in order to "gain" the benefits of exercise. You undergo the pain of denying yourself your favorite junk foods, in order to gain a slimmer, healthier body. A college student might sacrifice going out with her friends in order to gain the career benefits of good grades.

Self-denial and self-sacrifice are supposed to be good for us. They are supposed to bring physical, financial, and spiritual benefits. Work hard and save money now so you'll be able to enjoy a better future. Eat fewer calories now, so that you can have extra for dessert later. Sacrifice your own pleasures and desires, serve others instead, and you get to go to heaven. Go against the grain of selfish desires to build up karmic rewards.

A friend of mine once went on a seven-day Zen meditation retreat, at which talking and eye contact were prohibited. "How was it, Bill?" I asked. "It was torture," he replied. "It was hell. So I know it must have been good for me." What he meant is that seven days of practicing extreme self-discipline and restraint would strengthen his willpower, so that he would be better able to discipline and restrain his desires in the rest of life. He would be better able to make himself get up earlier, work harder, eat healthier, and so on. His spirituality was practice for more effective self-forcing.

This kind of spirituality is hard. It is an ordeal, an effort that never ends. It says, "Life is hard." It says, "All good comes from effort and sacrifice." That is why monks wore scratchy hair shirts and flagellated themselves. Similar practices still exist today. This idea that we must conquer the flesh for the sake of the soul points to the cultural origin of the war against the self, the war against pleasure, and the war against desire. I call it the second-oldest lie in the universe.

The second-oldest lie in the universe is that human beings are composed of two parts, a good part and a bad part. The good part is called the spirit, the soul, the mind, the civilized part, or the human part. The bad part is called matter, the flesh, the body, the instinctual part, or the animal part. Pleasure and desire, obviously, belong to the second part, the bad part. They arise from the flesh. To be good, then, means to conquer the flesh, to conquer the desires, and to deny oneself pleasure. That's supposed to be the way to goodness.

This is the root of the thinking that says bodily goodness, i.e. health, comes through controlling desire. Ultimately, it is the second-oldest lie that generates the child-rearing practices I described earlier. It says that children are born wholly uncivilized and selfish, pure creatures of desire, and we have to civilize them and train them not to just *do whatever they want*. This is a long story that I tell in depth in my other books, particularly *The Ascent of Humanity*.

For the present purpose, it is enough to see how pervasive this way of thinking is in our culture. All around us, so subtly we usually don't notice it, the message, "You are bad" and (therefore) that "You have to try hard to be good" is drummed into us. It is in our language, our way of thinking. Do you ever say something like, "It would have been really easy for me to just start shouting, but I was patient instead." The assumption here is that shouting is easy, patience is hard, and you have to fight an uphill struggle to be good. And what about that woman over there, yelling at her kid right now? Well, she just must not be trying as hard. Can you see the judgmentality built into hard-equals-good? I hear it all the time: "If so-and-so would at least make an effort..." It is the same kind of judgment people direct at your fatness. They think you're just not trying very hard.

Underneath such judgments is an implicit self-congratulation. I'm not overeating, I'm not shouting, because I'm being a good boy and trying harder. Mommy, where is my reward? Well, mommy isn't going to give you a reward any more, so instead you pat yourself on the back, allow yourself a bit of love—and maybe reward yourself with a few donuts. Underneath every judgment is an unmet need. Have compassion for all the people judging you for being fat. They are doing what they have learned to do to allow themselves a bit of self-love.

Here's another example of our belief in our inherent badness: why is the word "selfish" typically an insult? It would not be an insult if the self were fundamentally divine. It would not be an insult if we believed that pleasure and desire led us to greater goodness, kindness, and compassion. If selfish is bad, then struggle is necessary to overcome that bad self. This book offers an alternative to all of that.

What about trusting yourself so much that you are not afraid to be selfish? What about trusting the desires of your body so completely that you never think of denying yourself any food you want? This is the true freedom that I offer you in this book. With the concept of substitute desires, we are already one-third of the way there. Soon we will examine pleasure in the same way, to discover the true pleasure that leads to the fulfillment of our needs.

Before I do that, a word of warning... wait—are you prepared for me to tell you it is going to be hard? Anything truly good for you has got to be hard, right? To achieve goodness you have to fight against the grain of your natural desires. In that belief, we see the second-oldest lie in the universe rear its ugly head again. Transformation is supposed to be hard. If it comes easy, if it comes without sacrifice and struggle, it can't be very good, can it?

I ask you to let go of this belief. Because the path I lay out in these pages is not hard. It is easy. I am not going to let you validate it by making it hard. That would be the mentality of dessert. You no longer need to do something hard in order to allow yourself goodness. Health and happiness (and patience, and any other virtue) can come easy. Why? Because they are our birthright. They are our true nature. The natural tendency of the body is toward health, not away from it. To be obese is not your default state that you can only exit through struggle. Your true nature—vibrant health—wants to come out. It has been waiting a very long time. If you have read this far, it means you are ready to accept this. You are ready to relax into your true nature.

Chapter Nine

Substitute Pleasures

Let us return to that key question, "Why does it *seem* like the things that make us fat and sick are the things that give us the most pleasure?" It just seems so obvious: to lose weight, you're going to have to give up the things you love to eat the most. You're going to have to give up pleasure. It's going to be hard.

The answer to this riddle is related to the concept of substitute desires: the things we *think* give us the most pleasure actually do not give us the most pleasure. When we provide a substitute for a true desire arising from an unmet need, we are giving ourselves a substitute for the true pleasure we would get from fulfilling that need. In effect, we are substituting a lesser pleasure for a greater pleasure.

Usually, though, we are not aware that this is happening. We think we are giving ourselves more pleasure, not less, when we binge on our favorite food. We think we are indulging our desire for pleasure. This is an illusion, and I am going to tell you how to pierce that illusion.

The reason we think we get maximum pleasure by bingeing and overeating is that we actually do not feel most of the pleasure (and discomfort) available when we eat. In fact, I would say that most people experience less than one percent of all the sensations available from eating food.

Another way of putting it is that we actually do not know which foods we like. We think we know, but we do not. How could we possibly know if we don't fully taste and experience them?

Why don't we fully taste and experience our food? Usually, it is because our attention is on something else. Here is another truth that will never change: you can only pay attention to one thing at once. Play around with this idea and you will find that it is true. You might be able to switch your attention back and forth quickly to give the illusion you are paying attention to two things, but no being can pay attention to more than one thing at once, because in essence we *are* attention. I don't mean to get metaphysical here; the important point is that your real food at any given moment is whatever you are paying attention to.

That means if you eat in front of the television, you are actually feeding yourself the TV program. If you eat while feeling guilty, you are feeding yourself guilt. If you use food to create an emotional state of comfort, that is what you are feeding yourself. If you are eating donuts and focused on the emotional gratification that you use them to substitute for, then your body thinks that the donuts *are* the emotional gratification.

Only if you pay attention to what the donuts actually are, will your body understand that they are not self-love, not connection, not intimacy, not whatever they substitute for. When your body understands that, they will no longer work as a substitute, and the craving for them will disappear like magic. Similarly, when you fully experience the sensations of overeating, you learn *in your body* that you are not actually taking in self-love, or connection, or excitement, or any of the other things you use food for. You dissociate food from these other things. Food becomes only what it is. Food becomes food, that is all.

For this to happen, you must actually taste the donuts. You must fully, fully taste them, fully be present for the entire experience of eating them. How else can your body know them for what they are? The next time you sit down with your favorite binge food, take a few moments to smell and anticipate it beforehand. Then eat it with full attention and no distractions, bite by bite. After you are done, sit for a few minutes and feel the aftereffects of the food in your body.

You can never really know any food if you eat in front of the computer, on the phone, driving, reading, or watching television. All you can know of that food is the one percent or so that is intense enough to distract you from that other activity. That is why I say most people only taste one percent of their food. If they tasted the other 99%, they would make very different food choices indeed.

Think about the snack foods that are popular today. Their appeal lies in that 1% of the flavor that can break through the attention barrier. The surface taste is very intense, a result of artificial flavors, MSG, salt, sugar, spice extracts, and other additives. Underneath they are very empty and often repulsive, but we typically don't taste that part.

One of the most insidious distractions from experiencing food is mental dialog. For example, if you binge while thinking, "This is the last time. I'll never do this again. Starting tomorrow, I'm turning over a new leaf," then guess what? You will unconsciously associate the binge with the positive feelings of turning over a new leaf. You will accomplish the opposite of what you intend.

Even worse, by doing this you continue to program yourself for failure. You were using your binge food as a substitute for what you really wanted. The unmet need underneath will continue to drive your desire. Remember the pressure-cooker story. In the war against desire, desire always wins!

The way out of this trap is to let go of these internal distractions as well as the external ones, and purely and simply experience your food for what it is. Most importantly, you will have to let go of the guilt and shame that so often goes along with overeating. Ordinarily, we use guilt and shame as a whip to frighten ourselves into better behavior next time. In the case of bingeing and overeating, this strategy backfires. It exacerbates the need for love, comfort, and self-acceptance, causing yet more bingeing and more guilt in a vicious neverending circle. The *only* exit from the pattern is to identify and satisfy the true underlying need. And the pathway to the need lies through pleasure, again because of that unchangeable truth: it feels good to meet our needs.

When you put your attention just on the food, just on the physical sensations of eating, something amazing happens. Foods that do not really meet your needs start to give you less pleasure, and foods that harm your body begin to taste bad. It is a natural process—no effort or struggle is necessary. With highly processed foods and junk foods, you begin to experience that other 99% of the eating experience, the part I described as empty and repulsive. Then you no longer desire that food, because your natural desire is for pleasure.

In my seminars, we practice eating a bite of food, say a piece of apple, with full attention and full dedication to pleasure. People are amazed at how much pleasure, how rich an experience, is contained within a bite of an apple. Existence is a playground of delights. When we connect with this, we no longer starve for the pleasure that is so freely available around us. Now, I don't eat every bite of food this way, but once in a while I will eat a piece of food or even a whole meal with full attention and devotion to pleasure, just to reconnect and re-mind myself of the basic blissfulness of being alive. When we experience that, we escape the trap of desperately seeking pleasure while ignoring the pleasure available—a common pattern of food abuse.

This is the practical food application of the self-accep-tance we discussed earlier. It is to trust your natural desire for pleasure, and to trust that your body indeed gets the most pleasure from meeting real needs. You trust your body and accept its requests. You no longer fight desire or withhold pleasure. Instead, you come to a deeper and deeper under-standing of what you want and what feels good. You relax into freedom.

Chapter Ten

Killing the Pain

Once upon a time there was a man who had never experienced fire. One day he moved to civilization and saw his first hot stove. He thought it would be fun to touch the hot coil. Ouch! It really hurt. He certainly had no desire to do that again. Just like you, he didn't need to reason with himself, "I sure would like to, but I know it would cause tissue damage, open me to infection, and so on, so I guess I'd better not." Do you need to exercise willpower to stop yourself from pinching your own nose really hard? Do you need to exercise willpower to refrain from giving yourself a good hard poke in the eye? Of course not. It is our fundamental nature to avoid pain.

The man's brother, however, was not so fortunate. When he moved to civilization, a foolish anthropologist gave him a jar of anesthetic cream, "Just in case you hurt yourself," he said. The man put it on his hands and proceeded to touch the beautifully glowing hot stove. He didn't feel any pain until much later, when he'd forgotten he'd even touched the stove. He rubbed on some more cream—problem solved! Time went by and he kept touching hot stoves. Why wouldn't he? His hand hurt all the time and he didn't know why. All he knew was that he could get temporary relief from the anesthetic cream. But as the damage spread and gangrene set in, the cream became less effective. He moved on to stronger and stronger painkillers.

Because the man never had the chance to integrate the experience of pain with the act of touching the stove, he never learned in his body not to do that. As his problem got worse, he read all kinds of theories about why hands hurt. "This is bad for you, that is bad for you," they said. He tried to apply this knowledge to stop himself from doing various things, but how could he really be sure which was correct?

Most people in our society are much like this second brother. We are also told, "This food is bad for you, that food makes you fat, this food causes cancer, that food causes heart disease," but how can we know for sure? How can we know in our bodies, not just in our minds? How can we find the easy certainty we apply when we refrain from poking our-selves in the eye?

Eventually the second brother stopped using his anes-thetic cream and painkillers, and soon it became obvious why he kept hurting all the time. He'd read touching hot stoves was bad, but he'd never believed it until now. Now it really hurt! He no longer had any desire to touch them. The only willpower he needed was a gentle reminder, the mindfulness necessary to break an old habit you've outgrown.

Similarly, you already know in your head that overeating and sugar harm your body. You know it in your head, but not in your body. There is only one way to know it in your body, and that is to feel it. When you feel the full effects of a choice that generates pain, you will no more want to repeat that choice than you will want to poke yourself in the eye.

Unfortunately, our culture has conditioned us to be like the second brother in the story. Anytime we encounter discomfort or pain, our ingrained response is to do something to avoid feeling it. We go to the doctor complaining of pain, and are pleased to receive a pain-killer. Pain is not believed to have a positive purpose, so one goal of medical therapy is to find a way that it not be felt. We do the same with various forms of self-medication through drugs, addictions, and more subtle means. One way is to seek out some form of entertainment. When you entertain guests, you bring them into your home. When you entertain an idea, you bring it into your head. When you are being entertained, the television is bringing you out of yourself. The TV, the movie, the video game, or whatever absorbs your attention allows the pain or discomfort to go unfelt. Anything to make it feel better.

Of course, if there is a real wound generating the pain, then watching TV or eating a cookie or having a good stiff drink probably isn't going to heal it. What's more, an unhealed wound often gets more and more painful while the distraction gets less and less effective. This is the fundamental dynamic of addiction.

Any substance or activity is potentially addictive if it makes a wound temporarily stop hurting, but does nothing to heal that wound. Most addicts are hurting from deep wounds inflicted in childhood. In fact, I believe that in our culture all of us are wounded to some extent, and we are attracted to various addictions according to the nature of the wound.

The logic of addiction says that we can numb the pain of an unhealed wound forever. A series of temporary fixes can make us feel good indefinitely. Feel bad from too much dinner? Have dessert. Feel even worse? Have a smoke. Feel bad again five minutes later? Let's watch a DVD. Let's have a nightcap. On and on and on, an endless quest to escape the pain and feel good. It is quite understandable: all beings desire to feel good. There is fundamentally nothing wrong with the logic of addiction, except that it does not work. Its promise is a lie. I call it the "third-oldest lie in the universe": that we can avoid the pain without healing the wound. Well, as any addict who hits bottom will tell you, all the deferred pain will be waiting for you in the end.

Dependency alone is not enough to make something an addiction. We are, after all, dependent on breathing, but we are not addicted to breathing. Holding your breath is uncomfortable, it is true, but when you breathe again you are not merely distracting yourself from the discomfort. You are actually meeting the real need for oxygen. That is why you don't require an ever-intensifying dose of breath to feel good!

Food is the same way. If you eat food to meet the real need of the body for fuel, vitamins, minerals, fats, amino acids, and so on, you are not addicted to food. The type of discomfort that arises when these needs are not met is called "hunger". Pretty simple, isn't it? We eat and the discomfort goes away, because we are meeting the true need.

The situation is quite different with a food addiction. Here the need isn't for food at all, but we eat food anyway to feel good. Like a drug fix, it works for a while, but because the real need goes unmet, we soon feel bad again. Naturally, we do what worked last time: we eat more food! This is the classic vicious cycle of addiction. It is so powerful that many people will eat food to alleviate the discomfort caused by... eating too much food!

To repeatedly apply food, or any addiction, to make ourselves feel better temporarily is just like the brother constantly applying anesthetic salve to his burned hand, or the woman eating ice cream to assuage thirst. Not only is the underlying need unmet, but it also prevents us from discovering what that need is.

The things we do to keep the pain at bay not only fail to heal the wound underneath; they also make that wound tolerable. They perpetuate a wounded, hurting state of being. They drive a constant anxiety, a constant restlessness. There is no peace, because unfelt pain is always there, waiting for any undistracted moment to be felt. That is the origin of boredom—it hurts just to be. Do you ever eat because you are bored?

If it is true that numbing or deferring the pain perpetuates the wound, then might it also be true that feeling the pain could help us find and heal the wound? We have made an enemy of pain. Could it be that pain is actually an ally in healing? I believe that all parts of our being have a purpose. The next section will explain the purpose of pain, and how it can help you heal your body and transform your life.

Chapter Eleven

A Call for Attention

Once upon a time there was a woman who sat on a tack. By chance, it missed the nerve when it went in, but pretty soon it started to hurt. She didn't know why her posterior was hurting. It was very uncomfortable though, and soon the pain spread all over her backside. She began to hold her body in a different way and walk with a limp. Her whole body hurt all the time and she didn't know why.

She went to her doctor for help. "I hurt everywhere," she said. Her doctor gave her some pain medication, which helped for a while, but eventually even increased doses couldn't make her feel better. She asked her friends. They tried to cheer her up by taking her mind off it. "Let's go shopping!" said one. "Let's eat some donuts!" said another. "Let's have a drink!" said a third. But these solutions were just like the doctor's pain medication. As soon as the shopping trip was over and the donuts consumed, the woman felt just as bad as before.

Other friends, thinking themselves wise, offered all kinds of philosophical advice. "This too will pass," said one, "so just keep enduring." Another one said, "Your pain is the result of bad karma, and when you've worked it all off it will go away." A third friend said, "Life just hurts, it is the way things are. Detach from the pain and you will feel better."

Fortunately, this was a courageous and strong woman. She was fed up with being in pain all the time, just as you are fed up with being fat. And she refused to believe that life is just like that, just as you refuse to believe that obesity is your permanent condition. So one day she said, "Enough! No more escaping the pain. (After all, escaping isn't working any more anyway.) I give up. I'm just going to feel it."

She stopped trying to take her mind off it. She stopped trying to think of something else. She sat down and let herself just feel it and feel it and feel it. After all those years, finally she was giving the pain her full attention.

(That is what pain wants, you know. It wants your attention. If it does not get what it wants, it will ask more loudly.)

After the woman fully felt her pain for a while, she started to notice some things she'd never noticed before: many different sensations in different parts of her body that she'd all lumped together as "pain". We use that one word to encompass so much! She noticed an emanating source in her backside, surrounded by layer after layer of holding, tension, and compensation. "Aha!" she thought, "that's where it is coming from." Soon it became obvious. "I wonder if there is a tack in my butt?" she wondered. She reached around and pulled it out.

Pain has two main functions in the human being. The first I have already mentioned: it is to warn us that we are hurting ourselves. It is a message from some part of the body saying, "No! Don't do that."

The second function of pain is as a call for attention. Pain is your body's way to direct attention to a wound. There is a saying, "Energy flows where attention goes." Pain directs attention, and therefore healing energy, to the source of the hurting.

Figure 4: The Purpose of Pain

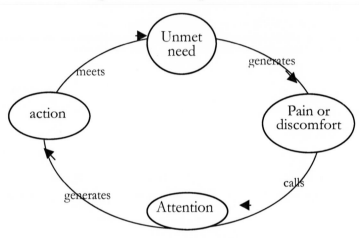

Pain is a call for attention to what is missing or to a wound that is hurting.

Even without any other action, attention is healing all by itself. You can feel that in the presence of a true doctor or healer—you feel better already. The same happens when a good friend truly listens to you. You haven't taken any action yet, but you feel better already. And, like the woman with the tack in her butt, the result of the attention is often a new kind of action, action that feels natural and right and not very difficult.

By avoiding the pain, you are avoiding healing. But please be careful to understand this correctly. I am not telling you to seek out pain. I am only telling you to listen to your body's messages. More deeply than that, what I'm really telling you is to BE. To feel what there is to feel.

Remember the pleasure principle: it feels good to meet our needs. But how can we accurately choose what feels good, if we haven't really experienced what feels bad? How can the second brother choose not to touch hot stoves, if he has never allowed himself to feel the burn? How can you choose not to overeat, if you don't allow yourself to fully feel the discomfort of overeating? How can you choose a different state of being, when you haven't fully experienced the one you are in?

The good news is that no matter how hard you try to stop it, the pain *will be felt*, one way or another, eventually. Many of you have reached that point already. There is no more escaping the various kinds of emotional and physical pain that accompany the state of chronic obesity. Now I am asking you to remove that last shred of resistance, and fully feel what it is like to be you right now. The same goes for every food choice you make. I will ask you to fully feel the results of every food choice you make. I will not require you to "do something about it." That is the path of control that hasn't worked. To simply feel will exercise a magical power.

The purpose of fully feeling the discomfort of a poor food choice is not to torture yourself. It is not a punishment for being bad. It is simply so you can integrate the results. Touch as many hot stoves as you want—but make sure to feel the results. Soon you will no longer desire to make those poor choices. You just won't want to. You won't have to apply mental threats to stop yourself. Because you want to feel

good. That is the simple truth that will revolutionize your relationship to food.

The goal here is pleasure, not pain. Pleasure and desire
are your friends, so make sure to fully feel pleasure as well. I
am asking you to pay more attention to your food. Many
overeaters think their problem is that they love food too
much. Actually the opposite is true—they do not love food
enough. An overweight woman recently told me how much
she enjoys drinking Coke. Nothing like relaxing in front of
her computer with an icy Coca-Cola, she says. But I don't
think it is really the Coke she likes. She likes that whole relaxing scenario. What would happen if she really tasted Coke?
Sip by sip by sip. She would discover that Coke isn't really
what she wants. She is using it to unlock something else: re-
laxation.

This book asks you to enjoy food more, not less. It asks
you to seek out every particle of pleasure food can provide.
You are going to get serious about loving your food. You will
realize that your body naturally wants to feel good, and that
your body knows how to do that. Obesity and sickness are an
unnatural state, a state maintained only by constant artificial
effort. This effort has become a habit—that's why it seems
that obesity is your default state. But now it is time to release
this lifelong habit of trying and forcing, and return to your
birthright of great health and fitness.

Chapter Twelve

The Three Mantras of Food Sanity

I have created three simple mantras to help you apply the principles we have explored so far. Together, they are a very simple, very radical way to totally reprogram your relationship to food. A mantra is a sentence that you repeat to yourself over and over again. I call these three principles "mantras" because they are so foreign to our ordinary way of thinking that you need to repeat them and work with them over time.

The most effective use of a mantra is to say it with full attention and understanding, so that you are repeating to yourself not just the words, but the meaning as well. However, even if you only repeat the words, mechanically, the meaning will gradually penetrate your consciousness on deeper and deeper levels. Also you will spontaneously discover new meanings, new understandings.

Notice again any fear response that arises as I describe the three mantras of food sanity. It may take the form of, "It is too good to be true." Only use them if you feel ready to trust them. If not, please wait until you are ready. Remember, you never need to force yourself to move beyond fear. When you are ready to take a step into the unknown, you will know that you are ready; you will be impatient for it. As you will see, these Mantras of Food Sanity are a step into the un-known. Trust your natural sense of caution and your natural desire to unfold and transform.

Mantra #1: "I give myself full permission to eat as much as I want."

Mantra #2: "I give myself full permission to eat whatever I want."

Mantra #3: "I take full pleasure in everything I eat."

Sounds pretty dangerous, doesn't it? So let me put these mantras into context so that you can apply them to your full benefit.

Mantra #1: "I give myself full permission to eat as much as I want."

You can also simplify it to, "I may eat as much as I want," or, "I'm allowed to eat as much as I want." Use what-ever works for you, whatever catches the spirit of this mantra.

What it means is that you sit down to a meal without any intention of limiting yourself. This should be a relief, since that intention doesn't really work anyway. Throughout the meal you continue to remind yourself, "As much as I want." At some point you'll start to get full and wonder if you should keep eating or if you should stop. Your ingrained habit will be to wonder, "Should I eat more? Should I stop? Is it OK to have another helping? Will it be too much? Is it justified? Is it good for me?" These are the habits you will now release. No more "should"! Instead you will simply ask yourself, "Do I *want* more?" Your task is to access true desire and trust true desire. Many of you have not eaten a meal like this in a very long time.

When you practice this over time, you cultivate a new habit of eating as much as you want. Under the regime of self-denial, we imagine that "as much as I want" equates to "as much as I can possibly stuff down my throat." That's the distrust of the self. We are trying out a different way now. You will discover that your true desire is not, in fact, to stuff yourself. When you give yourself full permission to eat as much as you want, your unconscious mind breathes a sigh of relief. You are giving yourself permission to no longer eat *more* than you want. Think about it. "As much as I want" means "no more and no less than what I want."

If you are an overeater and you practice this mantra, then over time you will discover something amazing. By giving yourself permission to eat as much as you want, you will start eating less, because you never really wanted all of that food. I bet that you have had this realization many times. "Why did I eat that?" you wonder. "I really didn't want it."

There are two levels of self-trust built in to this mantra. For one, you trust that your body indeed only wants the right amount of food. You trust that your body's natural tendency is toward health and not obesity. Secondly, you trust that you will know what this desire is. You trust that you will know when you have had enough, and you trust that you will naturally stop eating when you have reached that point. In other words, you trust desire, and you trust trust.

Let me warn you that if you pretend to use this mantra without actually using it, the results may backfire. If you secretly think, "OK, I will give myself permission to eat as much as I want, but only if it is no more than I think I should have," then you are not actually giving yourself total permission. If you monitor and evaluate your eating performance you will not actually be in touch with true desire. You will be experiencing the monitoring and evaluation, and not the actual food. The permission has to be total. You cannot fool your unconscious mind.

The fact is, you cannot "figure out" how much you actually want. You cannot use your mind to figure out the desire of your body. The body speaks its own language. The language of food-desire is hunger. If you pay attention, you will discover that there are many different sensations that we group under the word "hunger". Some of them are not really hunger at all, or at least not hunger for food. So another way to work with this mantra is to ask yourself during a meal, "Am I still hungry *for food*?" Let go of attachment to any desired answer. Maybe you are thinking, "I hope the answer is no, so that I will eat less and lose weight." It is important to be open to a Yes or a No, and to respect both. That is how to reestablish the authority of your authentic appetite for food. When you return authority to the authentic appetite, food will no longer be a substitute for other needs.

Only if you fully trust the Yes to "Am I still hungry for food" will you also easily and naturally trust a No. You are letting go of control and giving up on second-guessing yourself. It has not worked! Have you ever really tried self-trust over a period of time? Not the explosion of pent-up desire, but sustained self-allowing and self-trust? Perhaps not. Because in our society, to do that is such a huge step you could call it revolutionary.

Mantra #2: "I give myself full permission to eat whatever I want."

There are many people who very seldomly allow themselves to eat what they want. They have two ways of choosing food. In the control mode, rational criteria govern each food choice. "Is it good for me? How many calories does it have? Do I deserve it? Is it low-fat (or low-carb, or low-whatever)? Is it right for my blood type, my Ayurvedic type, my metabolic type?" Then there is the out-of-control mode, which is a reaction to the control mode. In the out-of-control mode we quit listening to those mental criteria, which is a positive step, but unfortunately neither do we listen to the real desire of the body. To return to the pressure-cooker metaphor, the steam is popping seams all over the place, but still not coming through the original opening that was blocked. The true desire has been pent up for so long that the wanting-force is uncontrollable.

When you give yourself full permission to eat whatever you want, you need to pause a moment before a food choice and ask yourself, "What food (if any) do I really want right now?" Don't worry too much about whether this wanting might be coming from a non-food need. Simply evaluate your choices at the moment. "Nothing at all" is always an option, or perhaps what you really want is a glass of water. (The displacement of non-food needs onto food sometimes causes people to eat when thirsty.)

Do not attempt to reason out what you think you *should* be wanting right now. Instead, feel the wanting in your body and ignore all those reasons and logic that justify or rationalize your choice. Again and again, say to yourself, "I can have whatever I want."

Just as with the first mantra, as you practice this over time you will find your tastes begin to change. You will discover that things you once wanted, or thought you wanted, are no longer attractive to you. And this will happen just by giving yourself permission to have what you want. No struggle is necessary.

The only effort you need to exert is to *remember*. Before you open the refrigerator or cupboard, remember to pause for that moment to feel desire in your body. This is for your benefit. You are doing yourself the favor of taking a moment to choose what you want the very most. In the out-of-control mode, we are like the woman who always orders the first item on the menu every time she goes to a restaurant. Take the time to peruse the whole menu, so you can choose the yummiest, most satisfying dish.

Visualize this mantra as a moment of luxury. All of these wonderful choices are before you, and you get to pick the very best one! You can have whatever you want! Don't waste this amazing opportunity by picking something you actually do not want. Why pick less when you could have more?

Even if you end up choosing a food that your reason and knowledge say is bad for you, don't worry. The immediate food choice is less important than the new habit you are cultivating. The habit is, again, self-trust. Each time you choose based on desire, without guilt or justification, you are sending yourself a message that you now trust yourself.

Mantra #3: "I take full pleasure in everything I eat."

Many people are so alienated from their bodies and from desire, that if you ask, "What do you really want right now?" they may say, "I think I want..." But thinking has nothing to do with wanting! You cannot deduce what you want, you can only feel what you want. But because our educational system and culture emphasizes thinking over feeling, we often attempt to think our way toward that which must be felt.

When you begin using the first two mantras, you may go through a period where you are often unsure about your true desire. That is OK. Clarity will grow with time. However, if you want to vastly accelerate this process, I suggest you also apply the third mantra: "I take full pleasure in everything I eat." This has two important and closely-related benefits. First, it will accustom you to pay attention to feeling, not thinking, when it comes to food. Remember, that mental knowledge about what and how much is "good for you" has never made much difference. You need physical knowledge, knowledge in the body where authentic desire comes from.

Secondly, this mantra will allow you to integrate in your body the consequences of your choice. If the choice was a good one, you integrate the pleasure and satisfaction that result. If the choice was a poor one, you integrate the discomfort. Next time, your desire will be much clearer in your body.

It is perhaps understandable that people try to avoid the experience of pain; what is more puzzling is that they often avoid the experience of pleasure as well. Often we don't take the time or devote the attention to fully enjoy the foods we like. Next time you eat a bag of candy, chips, or cookies, notice how your attention might be already on the next bite, or the next snack, before the present mouthful is even chewed. You are bypassing the actual pleasure of the food, which comes from the immediate sensation. The same is true if you eat while reading or watching TV.

Many people do this at a meal too. Next time you sit down to dinner, notice if your mind is already on dessert even before the first course if finished. This pattern is a sure sign that food is substituting for other needs.

When you don't fully taste food, your body doesn't really know what it is getting. No wonder you are confused when you try to decide what you really want! Not knowing the food for what it is, you naturally use it to substitute for other needs. But when you fully experience food, the illusion that it is actually self-love, excitement, self-expression, or connection is no longer tenable. Because now you know, in your body, exactly what it is and what it is not.

I have phrased this mantra in terms of pleasure, because that is what food will bring us when it meets our needs. However, you might want to rephrase it as something like, "I accept the full experience of everything I eat," because taking full pleasure in everything you eat also means experiencing all the unpleasurable feelings that come with food too. Your job is simply to feel. When you eat "whatever you want," make sure to feel any discomfort that may come afterward. In other words, listen to the echo of the food in your body after you eat it. Then, if that food wasn't meeting a true need, or is actually harming you, you will feel it. By paying attention to that feeling, you will integrate it. By integrating it, you provide yourself a solid basis for choosing next time.

Amazingly, having the full experience of food before, during, and after eating is *all* that is necessary to produce change. You don't have to accompany feelings of discomfort with an inner monologue of "Why did I eat that? Bad! I'll have to do better." Equally unnecessary is, "Let's see, is this bad feeling really coming from the food? How can I tell..."

All of that actually takes you away from the direct experience of the food. You don't have to figure anything out. All you have to do is feel. And make sure to feel the positive feelings too, of satisfaction and delight—even if they come from a food you think is bad for you.

People have a tendency to make this practice difficult. It is not difficult. It is so easy there is literally nothing to it. Anything you add onto it makes it less.

Let me emphasize again the importance of being present for the whole experience. As I explained earlier, typically if we feel bad as a result of a choice, we try to distract ourselves from the bad feelings. We could do it by having a smoke, popping in a DVD, entertaining fantasies about that being the last time: "I'll never do that again. I will not allow myself. I'm making a fresh start." Or, very often, we will distract ourselves from our discomfort by having something to eat.

It is time to release this habit. Eat whatever you want, eat as much as you want, and feel the whole process. If you overeat and feel bloated, stuffed, sluggish, foggy, and your tummy hurts, then sit and feel that, minute after minute after minute. Only then will you integrate on a body level what you are actually choosing when you overeat. Only then will you know how to choose pleasure in the future.

The medicine for food abuse is the results of food abuse. But like the woman who sat on a tack, you have to let yourself feel the results.

Even if you are afraid to apply the first two mantras, this third mantra of food sanity is powerful all by itself. If you apply it sincerely, you will awaken your natural body-wisdom and self-trust, and the first two mantras will become less scary with time. If you take only one thing from this book, let this be it. Be fully present for your food to obtain the most enjoyment possible from it. Ultimately, it is pleasure and joy that lead to health, because both health and pleasure are both aspects of our natural, true state of being.

Chapter Thirteen

Food Sanity in Action

Let me walk you through a scenario where you could apply all three of these mantras. Say you are hungry. "I can have whatever I want," you tell yourself, and there is a big bag of cookies. "I want those," you think. Maybe you don't have a clear sense in your body whether you indeed want them. No problem... let it go. You start eating the cookies, and fortunately you remember the third mantra. "I will take full pleasure in these cookies," you say. In order to do that, you give them your full attention, savoring every nuance. One, two, three... you eat cookie after cookie. Eight, nine, ten. You are committed to fully enjoying each one. "I can have as many as I want," you think. You finish the bag, and by now the good feelings in your mouth as you ate are fading away, and you tune into your body. You notice you don't feel very good. Not in your body, not in your emotions. You are full but not satisfied. You feel an ache, a cold loneliness, all kinds of emotions. And you just stay there with those feelings. You don't build a story around them to justify your choice or to blame yourself. You just sit and feel and feel and feel. That is all you need to do.

If you do this, I guarantee you that next time the cookies will be a less attractive choice. Without trying to stop yourself, you simply won't want them as much. And if you do eat them, you won't desire to eat as many. It may take a few times, but soon your body will have integrated what cookies really are. They won't be self-love or connection any more.

This is a great result, but please don't set it up as an expectation. Your job is simply to experience fully. The changes in your desires will arise naturally from that.

Do you get the amazingly good news in that sentence, "Without trying to stop yourself, you simply won't want them as much"? Yes, it can be that easy! Let go of the idea that transforming your life has to be hard. That idea has not served you well, but only brought you years of struggle. Trying hard has not worked. It is time to relax into freedom.

When you have used the Three Mantras for a while and gotten to understand, in your body, various foods and eating patterns, the Three Mantras will become more automatic, more just a part of who you are. I would like to describe an intermediate stage that sometimes occurs before food choices become fully aligned with true desire. To explain it, let's return to the bag of cookies.

Last time you ate the whole bag and felt terrible afterwards, but you have not integrated those feelings fully enough for the cookies to be as unattractive as a good hard poke in the eye. Today, you are feeling bored, lonely, or depressed, and there's another bag of cookies. This time you have more of a basis to know if they are what you want. Invoking the mantra, "I can eat whatever I want," you intentionally recall into your body the experience of eating them last time—not to try to figure out if you want them, but to provide yourself with a feeling-basis for choice. You recreate as best you can the experience of eating them, including the yummy sensations of crunching them in your mouth, as well as the bloated, unpleasant feeling of fifteen minutes after finishing them. Having walked yourself through all of the sensations, your body better remembers what the cookies are. You ask yourself again, "Do I want these cookies?" and you are open to any answer. You may choose to eat them, you may choose a glass of water or a walk or a nap instead; whatever your choice is, you allow yourself to fully experience and feel its results.

Eventually you will no longer have to go through this process. Your choices will be immediate and effortless. You can tell if you have genuinely made this transition by observing whether any of the following eight indicators hold true for you. If they do, it probably means that you are still using food to meet other needs.

1. I often eat when I am not hungry.
2. I am often not sure whether I am hungry or not.
3. I look forward to my next course, meal, or dessert while I'm still eating the one before.
4. Even when I've stuffed myself, I still want more.
5. My public eating and my private eating are very different. I like to eat special foods in secret.
6. I make and justify my eating choices on criteria other than hunger.
7. I evaluate my "food performance" and am pleased if I have controlled my eating today.
8. I often eat because I'm bored.

Finally, every person's habits of food abuse are different, and the negative beliefs associated with them are different as well. As you work with the Three Mantras, you can also adopt some other affirmations that address limiting thoughts and beliefs specific to your relationship to food, health, and the body. I provide some suggestions below, each of which embodies some of the concepts I've discussed so far.

Negative Attitude	Healing Affirmation
I cannot control my eating	I do not need to control my eating
My body is naturally fat	My weight is a perfect adaptation to my past.
I am greedy and overindulgent	I allow my true needs to be met
It is hopeless	I surrender to the new
I am confused and out of touch	I trust what feels good.
I don't know what is good for me	I trust pleasure and pain to guide me. Pleasure is the Yes of my body. Discomfort is the No of my body.
The changes I need to make are too big	I boldly do exactly what I am ready to do.
I am disgusting	I accept and release the way I am
What's wrong with me?	I accept and release my frustration
I hate my body	The fight is over

The pitfall in using affirmations is: do you really believe them? If you repeat them with a feeling of doubt, they will not facilitate change, and may even have the opposite effect. If you are fully ready for the change—and after reading this book, you very well may be—you will read the affirmation in a spirit of enthusiastic welcome. If you do feel doubt, then please work with them using the process in the next chapter. We don't want to stampede over any of our feelings, not even doubt or despair. They are part of who we have been, and any transformation starts there.

Chapter Fourteen

Reinventing the Possible

The state of your body is not an isolated aspect of yourself. It is connected to many other habits: habits of eating and exercising of course, and also habits of thinking, ways of seeing yourself, emotional patterns, expectations of how others will treat you, and beliefs about what is possible for your life. Put another way, you are deeply habituated to being fat. You are used to it. It is a familiar way of being.

Because being fat is connected to so many other things about you, much else is going to change along with your weight. In many important ways, you are becoming a different person.

Have you ever experienced a tragedy or piece of great fortune in your life, and thought, "I can't believe this is happening"? When we grow used to a given reality, we begin to think that nothing else is possible. Our subconscious mind thinks it will never change.

What happens if you change your way of eating while still maintaining all the other habits of fatness? Very likely, the diet will eventually return to alignment with everything else about you. Fat-associated emotions, expectations, and habits are part of a whole self that includes being overweight. Many of them are automatic, perhaps even invisible to you. They are programmed in at a very deep level. That is why I would like to offer you a way to reprogram your subconscious mind with a new reality-picture, a new knowledge of what is possible.

One way to reeducate your subconscious mind is to create a multi-sensory "picture" of the new reality you want to move into. The title of this reality might be something like, "I am slim, strong, and vibrantly healthy," or, "I look and feel great." Do not worry if this statement contradicts the facts right now. It is just the title of a story you will tell your subconscious mind. The subconscious will tune into the reality of any story you tell it, just as you can be absorbed in a storybook or film. Rationally you know it is not real, but right now you are communicating with the part of yourself that thinks it is real. That's the part you need to educate, because that's the source of all the unconscious habits of fatness.

Make sure to phrase the story title in the present tense. You don't want to program yourself with the reality-picture of weight loss always being something in the future.

Once you have a title, create as many sensory elements as possible of the new story of who you are. For example, make pictures in your head of what your body will look like. Create an image of looking down at a scale readout displaying your target weight. Be very detailed and specific, including an actual number. See yourself shopping for new clothes. What will they look like? Picture as vividly as you can the size tag. Make aural "images" as well. Hear people saying, "Wow, you look great! How did you do it?" Hear your own inner voice speaking too, maybe in conjunction with that image of a slim you in the mirror, saying, "I look great!"

To complete the story, attach to it the emotions you associate with being thin. Feelings of pride, accomplishment, confidence, optimism, excitement, and freedom might go along with the sounds and images you have created. As vividly as possible, immerse yourself in the new reality.

While you do this, stay simply with the story you have created. Don't put attention on rational arguments for why it could or couldn't happen. Do not put attention on hope or on doubt. Just for now, let the whole picture—sights, sounds, feelings—be completely real to you.

Repeat this exercise every day, even twice a day, and really enjoy the deliciousness of it. That deliciousness will motivate your subconscious mind to make the shift into that reality.

I want to emphasize again: the purpose of this is not to convince yourself that it is possible to be thin. It is not a form of persuasion. If you fall into persuasion mode, you'll come up with lots of reasons why it is *impossible* too. Besides, the subconscious mind does not pay attention to logic. To reeducate it, you have to draw it into as vivid a story as possible.

After you have finished, say to yourself, "I fully accept this new vision for my life." Well, well, is that statement really the truth? Maybe it isn't. Maybe part of you isn't quite ready to accept it. In that case, you will have an emotional response to the above affirmation, probably involving feelings of doubt, frustration, or despair. If your response is anything but enthusiastic affirmation—yes!—then there is still a bit more work to do to ready your whole self for transformation. Lying to yourself will not get you anywhere. All emotions are messages from the soul, messages from yourself to yourself about the stories and beliefs you hold. They are to be respected, not ignored or fought. That's part of the self-trust this book is about. Self-trust includes the *whole* self, even the "negative" emotions of fear, anger, apathy, and despair.

If any of these come up when you affirm your acceptance of being light, I invite you to take another step in the self-reeducation process. Here is what to do. When the negative emotion comes up, dive into it fully. Really go there. It is part of your condition, and you need to complete it before you will be truly ready to move on. To complete it means to feel it to completion. So give yourself a few quiet minutes to really feel the frustration, doubt, or hopelessness—one hundred percent of it. Stay with the intensity of the feeling, minute after minute, until it peaks and then gives way to something else. At that moment you will experience a shift— you will recognized it when it happens. You need not and cannot make it happen. It just will. It's not about trying, it's about being there for it.

When these emotions are completed, they will have served their function and will depart. Such is the lifespan of all beings! Ironically, in the past you may have prevented the emotion from reaching its full intensity by having something to eat to distract yourself. But today you are taking a new step of courage. You are dedicated to feeling fully and being fully alive. Soon, your body will change shapes to embody that new vitality.

After the negative emotion has peaked and shifted, it will give way to a positive emotion such as confidence, serenity, or euphoria. Spend a few moments, maybe half a minute, just enjoying this feeling and associating it with your story-picture of being thin.

In those few moments, if you find yourself cycling back to doubt, frustration, etc., it means you need a few more sessions for that emotion to be completed. You could continue sitting with it now and go through the process again, or you can save it for later. Be patient. You have been in the state of fatness for a long time. Let the transition be gentle and graceful.

I guarantee that after a few reeducation sessions like this, the negative emotions triggered by your acceptance of being slim will dissipate. Once might be enough, because you are ready for something new. Or it might take four or five sessions. The Three Mantras of Food Sanity are already such a powerful reversal of fat-person thinking that your subconscious mind will be unusually receptive to new patterns. Just by using the mantras, you are already rocking your world. The time for transformation is here!

I leave you with a brief summary of the reeducation process:

1. Create a title for the story of a new, lighter you.

2. Create a multi-sensory picture with concrete visual and auditory details.

3. Bring into your body the feelings you associate with success in achieving that picture.

4. Affirm: "I fully accept this for my life."

5. If any negative emotions come up, be with them until they peak and shift.

6. Integrate the good feelings that replace those negative emotions.

Chapter Fifteen

Real Food

The human body normally has a minimum requirement for a number of vitamins, minerals, amino acids, calories, fatty acids, and myriad other substances in order to function optimally. If any are in short supply, the body will generate a desire for something to fulfill that shortfall.

In a natural setting, where a variety of nutritious foods are available and where human beings are sensitive to body messages, these nutritional needs are easily met. The person will know exactly what she is hungry for. We see this in wild animals, who will sniff out just the right medicinal plants when they are sick, and just the right food plants high in minerals that they are lacking. If you asked them how they knew to eat that plant, they might say, "I was hungry for that."

Modern human beings have lost much of this sensitivity, with the result that we don't know what we are hungry for. Earlier we discussed the futility of eating more and more food to meet our need for love, connection, excitement, or self-expression. Well, it is equally futile to eat more and more food to meet a nutritional need that food cannot provide. For the principles of this book to be truly effective, it is therefore helpful to reconnect to what I call "real food".

If you follow the three mantras of food sanity and you don't have real food in your diet, here is what will happen.

You will feel truly hungry, and you will have full inner permission to eat whatever you want, but none of the choices before you will be very appealing or satisfying. "I am hungry but I don't know what to eat," you will say. That is why it is necessary to expand your food horizons to include foods that can meet your body's true needs.

One reason that wild animals do not overeat is that their diets are nutrient-dense. Wild plants typically have many times more vitamins and minerals than domesticated plants. I believe the flesh of wild animals is also more nutritious than that of domesticated animals. The only truly obese wild animal I have ever seen was a raccoon that frequented a state park campground. I think I was ten years old. I looked out of the tent and saw him, an enormous, fat raccoon, eating our entire bag of marshmallows and then a dozen eggs.

What would happen if you tried to meet your body's nutritional requirements by only eating marshmallows and eggs? Well, even though the eggs provide many important nutrients and the marshmallows provide plenty of calories, important vitamins and minerals would be almost completely missing. You wouldn't get any Vitamin C, for instance. No matter how much you ate, your body would say, "I'm not satisfied yet." And your body would continue being unsatisfied no matter how many eggs and marshmallows you ate.

Such is the case with the standard American diet. Out of habit, out of ignorance, out of convenience, the menu of choices on most people's plates cannot possibly meet their true needs.

I believe that nutrition is a science in its mere infancy. Nutritional scientists have identified a mere handful of essential vitamins and minerals, probably less than a hundred. The true number is probably in the thousands. Most of the essential vitamins, minerals, fatty acids, amino acids and so on were discovered through the deficiency diseases that happen when one is missing. But these hundred or so substances are a tiny fraction of the tens of thousands of biologically active chemicals to be found in nature. Perhaps most of them are not "essential" in the sense that its absence causes a recognizable deficiency disease. The body can usually compensate for a missing substance by converting other substances. The body is very resourceful. But this compensation comes at a cost. When the diet is depleted of biochemical richness, health begins to deteriorate. Immunity weakens, teeth decay, bones thin, organs and systems break down. The cause is not a single missing substance; there is not a single cause at all but a constellation of causes.

Ultimately, as you implement the ideas of this book, you will naturally gravitate toward real food. It will taste better to you, more satisfying. It will become what you naturally want. When you eat real food, your nutritional needs will be met with normal portions. You will not still feel hungry when you are full.

Many people are so accustomed to the standard American diet they hardly know what real food tastes like. Even the most natural items in a supermarket, the items along the outer perimeter (fruit, vegetables, meat, fish, cheese, dairy) are but a shadow of their former selves.

Consider fruits and vegetables. USDA statistics over the last half-century show a dramatic decline in the vitamin and mineral content of common fruits and vegetables since the widespread adoption of chemical agriculture. Mostly because of the gradual depletion of soils, some items have only ten percent the nutrient content of the food our grandparents ate as children. But you don't need Department of Agriculture scientists to tell you this. You can taste it. The bland, insipid taste of a supermarket strawberry or tomato tells you that it is not a vibrant food. Compare it to a garden tomato or a strawberry just picked, still warm from the sun, bursting with vitality. Now that's living! That is the food we were meant to eat. That is the food we still crave. Those are the vivid flavors that reaffirm our connection to nature, and that make us feel alive.

When we eat dead food, picked weeks or months ago, processed by enormous machines, adulterated with chemicals, shipped in refrigerated containers across continents, packaged into cans and boxes, then we feel as dead as the food is. But we crave life! We are beings of flesh and blood, with an irrepressible urge to be alive and feel alive and participate fully in the living world.

Simply to feel alive, we overeat more and more dead food just to extract the tiny amount of vitality that still remains in it. But the life in a box of breakfast cereal, a fast-food burger, or a bag of potato chips is so anemic that no matter how much we eat, we still don't feel alive. We eat vast quantities of it, and feel at best half-alive. But it is all that is available, so we eat more and more.

What makes real food unavailable? In a sense it *is* available; what makes it unavailable is culture, habit, ignorance, and economics. For example, organic produce has more nutrients and more flavor than chemical produce, but even organic vegetables are far less nutritious than the wild plants from which they were bred. Free-range meat is more nutritious than factory-farmed meat, but not as intense in flavor or nutrition as wild game.

Fortunately, to get back to real food doesn't mean going back to a Stone Age diet. If you want to lose weight and recover vibrant health, the most important transition is toward food that looks and feels like something that comes from nature. Locally-grown, fresh, organic food is best of course, but even the conventionally-grown, over-domesticated produce in the supermarket is a hundred times more alive than what you find in boxes, cans, and microwave-ready packets. This already is a tremendous step toward real food that can transform your body.

Because we crave the vibrancy and intensity of life, the bland, dead food of a standard American diet is enhanced by a variety of phony additives that simulate the intense flavor and appearance of real food. If you want to recover food sanity, I strongly recommend that you completely eliminate them from your diet. Read package labels and eliminate anything with the following substances:

- MSG (monosodium glutamate)
- Artificial flavors
- Artificial colors
- Aspartame
- Sorbitol, sucralose, and other artificial sweeteners
- Autolyzed yeast extract
- Hydrolyzed protein (usually soy protein)
- Spice extracts
- Preservatives and other chemicals with unrecognizable names

- "Natural flavors" (usually quite unnatural)
- Partially hydrogenated oil
- High-fructose corn syrup

You might notice that except for the last two items, none of these are major sources of calories. The purpose in eliminating them is to reconnect you with real food. That is what will help you lose weight. Reconnected with real food, your needs will be met without eating huge quantities. Your body will no longer want to eat to excess (at least not for nutritional purposes).

When you strip away the artificial additives, the high-tech processing, and the complicated combinations of ingredients, you are much better able to recognize food for what it is. You know what you are getting. Your body instinctively recognizes it. Food becomes food, and is less able to serve as a substitute, either for emotional needs or other nutritional needs.

The packages and cans, the artificial this and processed that, the fast food and the soda pop of the standard American diet cannot possibly nourish a human body. Obesity is written right into the menu as an accompaniment to every dish. No one is forcing you to eat these foods, but the power of culture and habit is considerable. In whole or in part, you will be withdrawing from American food culture and the obesity that goes along with it.

To reconnect to real food, use only natural, recognizable ingredients in your cooking. Stay away from powders and mixes composed of more than one ingredient. Herbs and spices are fine, but not soup mixes or protein powders. Your body does not recognize such things as food. I am even suspicious of the green powders and food bars for sale in health food stores. This advice applies especially to weight-loss powders. Absent the cues of deliciousness, texture, chewing, and satisfaction, your body does not recognize them as food. You finish your protein drink and you may feel full, but you feel empty too and you want some real food.

Some Examples of Real Food

- Fresh vegetables

- Fruit

- Seafood

- Meat

- Eggs

- Olive oil

- Butter

- Coconut oil

- Whole grains in whole form (rice, oatmeal, corn, buckwheat, etc.)

- Wholegrain or sourdough bread

- Mushrooms

- Sea vegetables

- Potatoes, yams, squash

- Water

- Unpasteurized milk

- Cheese

- Plain yogurt

- Nuts
- Beans
- Honey
- Molasses
- Real maple syrup

Some examples of fake food

- White bread
- All store-bought pastries, donuts, cookies, cakes, pies, etc.
- All soda pop (including diet soda!!!)
- Candy
- Fruit juice from a can or carton
- Pasteurized milk
- Chips, crackers, junk food
- Ice cream
- Commercial salad dressing
- French fries and other deep-fried foods
- Anything with the fake food substances listed above (MSG, corn syrup, etc.)

If you compare store-bought orange juice with juice that you squeeze yourself, you will understand what I mean by real food. You can really taste the superior vitality in the fresh-squeezed juice. The difference is remarkable. The human body is meant to eat foods that are fresh and vibrant, direct from nature. That is what we instinctively recognize as food. The farther removed the food is from nature, the more of it we need to feel fed.

You can see that reconnecting with real food requires a big change in your buying, cooking, and eating habits. When you follow the above guidelines and stay away from phony ingredients, practically the whole supermarket is off-limits. If there is any bad news in this book, this is it. You are looking at a radical life-change, that will go along with your radical body-change. The good news is that within the domain of real food, anything is allowed and you don't have to restrict portions. The reconnection to real food and real nourishment, physical and emotional, will automatically result in smaller portions.

Real food meets real needs. When real needs are met, desire is satisfied. It is just that simple.

The suggestion to return to simple, real food does not contradict the principle of "I give myself full permission to eat whatever I want." You are merely exposing yourself to a new menu of possibilities, and clearing your perceptions so that you are better able to sense what you actually want. I believe, though, that the idea of real food appeals to most of you already. In our culture of artificial environments, media images, and general phoniness, we all thirst for authenticity. More than any nutritional reason, that is perhaps why we feel so instinctively drawn to real food. We want to get real!

Chapter Sixteen

Expanded Horizons

Despite all I have written about trusting inner authority, external information about diet and nutrition can still be helpful. Even if a lot of that information is contradictory, it would be arrogant to dismiss out of hand the vast accumulation of knowledge from science and tradition. There are many wonderful books and teachings out there today that can point you toward new things to try. They are not a substitute for inner authority, but they can be a map to guide your exploration of new foods and new approaches to food. Indeed, you may be so habituated to fake foods, and so cut off from your body, that your progress will be much faster with some outside help.

Be mindful, though, that the suggestions I am about to offer are to show you new territory, and not to answer the question "What should I eat?" If you've read this far, you know that the answer to this question is unique for each individual. What's more, you understand the peril in the word "should": it is not external rules that will lead you to the perfect diet, it is your own authentic appetite, sensitivity, pleasure, and desire.

How will you know whether a given dietary approach is right for you? Your body will tell you by feeling great! Not only will you lose weight, but you will feel more energetic, your mood will improve, and you will feel less foggy, groggy, mucous-y, and constipated

A basic observation of this book is that fat people are usually malnourished. Often, the needed nourishment is of a type that cannot come from food: the need for connection, love, excitement, and so on. At the same time though, fat people usually suffer a corresponding malnourishment in a nutritional sense as well. The concept of substitute desires comes into play again. We might eat a lot of the wrong kind of food as a substitute for a little of the right kind of food. We keep eating and eating what we don't actually need, in hopes of finding what we do need.

One example of this is the consumption of vast quantities of low-fat foods. The human body has a certain need for fats and oils in the diet. Moreover, fat is a major trigger of the satiety mechanism that tells you you've had enough. If you eat a single "hearty portion" of one of those packaged low-fat meals, you are not going to feel very satisfied. You might need to eat four or five portions, thereby consuming a huge number of calories just to obtain the fat that meets your needs and makes you feel full.

Many people have found, seemingly paradoxically, that adding more fat to their diet helps them lose weight. Actually, there is no paradox. Not only is fat satisfying, but it can raise the metabolism and help the body burn hotter. Coconut oil in particular has received a lot of research demonstrating its metabolism-raising effects. Fat also helps moderate the effects of high-glycemic foods, providing a steady source of energy over many hours, and thus reducing the urge to binge and snack.

Fatty foods often taste delicious too. Remember, we are following a path of self-trust, and that includes trusting the feeling of satisfaction and well-being we might get from eating high-fat foods. On the other hand, if you eat too much rich, fatty food, your body will give you an unmistakable signal. You will get grossed out. It isn't hard to overeat a vast amount of carbohydrates, but if you binge on pure butter you probably won't be able to eat very much before you want to throw up.

You may think that fat and cholesterol will give you heart disease or some other problem. Actually, this claim is very dubious scientifically. A multibillion-dollar industry rests upon this "lipid hypothesis" of heart disease, and the research that contradicts it is often marginalized or misinterpreted. I won't go too much into the science here; if you are interested check out www.cholesterol-and-health.com, Uffe Ravnskov's *The Cholesterol Myths*, and Gary Taubes' New York Times article "What if it's all been a big fat lie?" and book *Good Calories, Bad Calories*. These resources can reassure you that your body's desires are not actually dangerous.

Ultimately, I don't think we need scientists to tell us how much fat, protein, starch, etc. to eat. Our bodies will provide us much more precise information—information specific to the unique being that each of us is. I use books on diet and nutrition simply as tools to open my horizons to new foods and ways of eating that I would never have thought to try myself. I will introduce some of my favorite resources, but be forewarned: all of them contradict each other in some way. You aren't going to find any agreement on "the answer" out there. Luckily, you don't need to get the answer from "out there" and you don't need to figure it out intellectually. These books are just to guide you in exploring what might be right for your unique body.

A personal favorite of mine is Sally Fallon's *Nourishing Traditions*, which describes traditional health-giving diets interspersed with delicious recipes and revealing exposés of the degeneration of our food system. Sally Fallon is a controversial figure in the nutrition field, and I am not qualified to determine whether her work is more scientifically sound than that of her detractors. I recommend it to you for two reasons. One is just my personal experience. For an important period of my life this book deeply resonated with me and led me to truly nourish myself for the first time in years. The second reason it is relevant to this book is that *Nourishing Traditions* is a clarion call for a return to real food. It opens our horizons to the variety of real foods that were once common, and explains how to prepare them.

Because overweight people are typically overfed and undernourished at the same time, the journey of returning to your healthy weight therefore is likely to involve periods of reducing and cleansing as well as periods of nourishing and rebuilding. *Nourishing Traditions* might helpful for the latter phase. For the reducing/cleansing phase, I recommend investigating various books advocating macrobiotics, raw foods, fasting, juicing, and sprouting. You can explore these and see if any resonate with your intuition and the sensory feedback of your body.

A dietary approach that is effective for this phase of weight loss is Donna Gates' *Body Ecology Diet*. It aims to restore the optimum acid-base balance in the body as well as a healthy intestinal flora by eliminating foods that create acidity and feed pathogenic yeasts. Her recipes emphasize eliminating gluten and dairy from the diet, substances that can be congesting for many people, and adding cultured and fermented foods and supplements. Significantly from the perspective of this book, she does not require limiting portions. Real food in the right combination leads naturally to weight loss without the constant battle against calories. I especially recommend Gates' book to people who suffer any kind of candidasis, allergies, or autoimmune disease. For many people, just eliminating gluten and dairy has a profound effect.

There are several nutritional schools of thought today that meet the issue of individual variation head-on. They attempt to explain and categorize the ways in which each person is unique. Some of these systems, such as Ayurveda and Traditional Chinese Medicine, are thousands of years old; others draw from modern biochemistry and physiology. Going by the general name of metabolic typing, the modern approaches are, I believe, still in their infancy as sciences. Some of the popular books on the subject include books on metabolic typing by William Wolcott and Dr. Joe Mercola; I have also gained many insights from the more technical work of Dr. Guy Schenker. Again, these systems have numerous contradictions among them, but they can help guide you toward something that works in your body. They explain why a high-carb diet works for some people and high-protein works for others, why some people do fine with nightshades and others do not, why certain vitamin and mineral supplements help some people tremendously and have little or negative effect on others.

These findings would not be surprising to a traditional Chinese doctor or Ayurvedic practitioner. These systems (and, according to Matthew Wood, pre-modern Western medicine as well) used herbs and foods not as one-on-one treatment for symptoms (this for headaches, that for constipation), but to rebalancing underlying bodily disharmonies. Thus, watermelon might be a perfect food for someone with a hot, dry constitution, and terrible for someone who is pale, bloated, and tending toward coldness. If you are interested in learning about the implications of these systems for diet, I recommend the work of the herbalist Michael Tierra for its attempt to synthesize Ayurvedic, Chinese, and Western systems.

Another powerful book based on Ayurveda that champions a return to real food is Gabriel Cousens' *Conscious Eating.* Although it advocates vegetarianism for everyone, a position I disagree with, it contains marvelous insights on the psychology and spirituality of food and food abuse. If you feel drawn to be a vegetarian, this book is an excellent resource. However, in order to get a balanced perspective, I also recommend reading *Nourishing Traditions* and my own book, *The Yoga of Eating.* I would also like to take the present opportunity to make a few more remarks about vegetarianism.

A surprising number of people adopt a vegetarian diet in part because they think it will help them lose weight. It may be their main motivation, or kind of an "added bonus" to its supposed ethical and spiritual virtues. But in fact, vegetarian diets sometimes have the opposite effect: weight gain. This is something I have noticed in my food activism over fifteen years, and I can also offer some scientific speculations as to why this happens. It could be because lower protein intake fails to sustain blood sugar levels, resulting in hunger. It could be because lower fat intake fails to trigger satiety mechanisms, resulting in overeating. It could be because an excess of soy depresses thyroid function, slowing the metabolism and promoting weight gain. While some people do lose weight on a vegetarian diet, at least initially, others gain weight. It is certainly no panacea.

From the perspective of this book, there is only one reason to become a vegetarian: if that is the flowering of your natural desires that gives you pleasure in your body. Many people do it for other reasons: to allow themselves self-love, to think of themselves as good, to be in accord with certain spiritual teachings. I say: What about loving yourself no matter what? What about not needing to establish yourself as good in your own eyes? I suggest putting everything on your menu of possibility. "I can eat whatever I want." That is full self-trust, full affirmation of your innate goodness. Just as your authentic desires will not bring you to fatness, neither will they bring you to evil. Spirituality is not a struggle against evil, and it is not a struggle against desire or pleasure. Remember: who is the loser in the struggle against the self? You are. The time has come to let go and trust.

I would like to tell you about one more book that is deeply aligned with these concepts: *The Diet of Now*, by the nutritionist Karine Rogers. Beautifully constructed in the form of a multi-course meal, this small book takes you back to the reality of the body again and again. It also contains practical tips on conscious eating, menu plans, and recipes. It is an excellent resource for weight loss.

In addition, there are literally thousands of alternative health sites on the Internet. Many of them are not very scientific, but I believe each offers at least a tiny window on the truth. There are sites advocating low-carb, low-fat, or low-protein diets. There are sites advocating diets for your blood type, your ethnic background, your Ayurvedic type. There are sites advocating various herbs and supplements. There are sites advocating fasting, juicing, and sprouting. I believe that all of them, even the most extreme, have some insight to offer. However, for most people all that information adds to the confusion and takes them out of the body and into the head. Knowing about food is not the same as knowing food. Knowing food only happens in the body. It cannot happen through reading. So let reading be maybe ten percent of your quest for health, something that points you toward new experiences, feelings, and body-knowledge.

Only your body knows what is the perfect program for you. If you, like most obese people, are overfed and undernourished at the same time, your body might lead you through a succession of phases where cleansing and reducing alternates with nourishing and rebuilding. You might go through days, weeks, or even months where all you want is fruit and salads, or brown rice and beans. Then you might want seafood, or steaks and hamburgers, or buttered yams. Can you accept that you don't have to *figure out* what is right at any given time? Figuring out means understanding it in your head. That is nice of course, but it isn't necessary for health. Does a deer "figure out" which plants are medicinal when it needs healing? No, it is simply attracted to those plants. Do chimpanzees, which have at least five times the strength of humans, "figure out" the ideal exercise and diet program? Of course not. They are simply in tune with their bodies. These capabilities are latent in human beings as well. Expand your sense of the possible!

You might be attracted to the high-protein Atkins-type diets that are extremely effective to initiate weight loss. Many people say of these, "It worked great for a while, but I couldn't stick with it." The same happens to many people on raw foods or vegan diets. You are not meant to struggle your whole life to "stick with" anything. Extreme diets might be beneficial for a while, but that doesn't mean they are perfect for a lifetime. Always let your body's responses guide you.

I am not going to offer you recipes in this book. Others have done that much better than I can! The reference books I have listed contain many great real-food recipes, and you can find more in any conventional cookbook. Just be sure to prepare dishes consisting only of real foods. Don't be afraid of high-fat or high-calorie dishes that you might think to be off-limits. Those days are over. Dieting hasn't worked, remember? You can eat whatever you want. Don't even think about calories; think about real food and most of all, follow your sense of what is delicious and nourishing. You will not lose weight by nourishing yourself less. In the new view, you can be good to yourself. "I can have whatever I want."

In the same spirit, remember not to limit your portions. The only limit is when it no longer feels good. "I can have as much as I want." You are allowing yourself the pleasure of fully feeding and nourishing yourself. You are trusting that with a return to real food, you will also return to your natural, authentic appetite and body wisdom. Both are rooted in nature. They *are* nature. The same goes for your body: its true nature is to be active, healthy, and fit. Your cells desire it, your organs desire it, your stomach, your brain, even your fat cells desire to be part of a smoothly functioning, vibrantly healthy organism. When you return to nature in all realms, the nature of the body's innate health will manifest as well.

As long as you trust yourself to choose from a variety of real foods, you don't have to worry. Your cellular wisdom will lead you through the ideal program to health. Eat whatever real food you want. Eat as much as you want. And allow yourself the full experience of whatever you eat.

The Three Mantras of food sanity will naturally lead you toward real food anyway. Your transition to healthy body weight will be much faster, though, if you start exploring a switch to real food right now. Make a variety of simple, natural foods available to help reset your body sensitivity and feed your real simple, natural needs.

Chapter Seventeen

Movement without Workouts

Modern adult human beings are the only beings in Creation that do workouts. Babies, children, primitive humans, and animals never do exercise just for the sake of exercise. They move their bodies either to perform necessary functions of life, or to play.

Guess who is healthier: modern adults who try to work out every day, or pre-technological people who only moved their bodies for work or fun? Primitive people were far more physically fit than we are today.

Your body is designed to be used. The muscles, bones, tendons, and nervous system exist in large part to move the body. It is part of your nature to be in motion. It is also a deep physical need. Again, a fundamental truth is that it feels good to meet your needs. Movement ought therefore to be a pleasure, not a burden. Obviously, something is amiss with the concept of a workout.

The concept of a workout is really quite new. On the face of it, it is rather silly. Riding an exercise bike that goes nowhere, walking on a treadmill for an hour to end up at the same spot where you started, lifting huge weights up and down without moving anything... it is all quite like digging a hole and filling it up again. A pointless, useless expenditure of time and energy. In fact, when you work out to burn calories, that is the whole idea. You are burning excess energy for no real purpose except to burn it.

Here is the single most important exercise concept for weight loss: *The purpose of exercise is not to burn calories.* Whether it is limiting your caloric intake or motivating yourself to burn more calories, the days of self-forcing and control are over. Life need not be an endless struggle to burn more calories than you take in.

Let me say it again. The purpose of exercise is not to burn calories. The purpose is to experience the joy of movement. Then your body will naturally tend toward a state that permits movement to happen. When you call upon your body to move, your body will reshape itself to facilitate movement. When you call upon your muscles to move, your muscles will grow. It actually requires an enormous amount of calories to grow new muscle, and the new muscle itself requires constant fuel to maintain itself.

If you are active, your body will tend toward a shape fit for activity. The question, then, is what is keeping you from being active? What is preventing the expression of your natural, inborn joy of movement?

If you have been on the weight loss treadmill for a long time, it may be "exercise" itself—the concept of the work-out—that is blocking the joy of movement. You will find that when you let go of exercising to burn calories, many forms of fun movement become available to you. You no longer have to worry about how long you do it or how many calories you burn. Any form of movement is acceptable.

Choose anything that gives you joy and pleasure. Some of the best forms of exercise are gardening, Tai Chi, yoga, dance, walking, and any kind of sport or physical game. Whatever you choose, find delight in it. If you walk, make sure you aren't only walking for exercise. Walk in nature, fill your senses with the sounds of insects and birds, and walk as fast or as slowly as you want to. If you take a dance class, don't do it for exercise. Find one that is fun and exciting on its own merits.

Exercise should be a side-effect of being alive, and not a separate maintenance activity. You may find that you enjoy traditional "workout" types of exercise such as swimming, running, or biking. I do a bit of all three myself, but only because it feels good, and I only do them when I want to. My running mostly happens in a playground with children. There is never a "should".

If you are immersed in workout mentality, you might even benefit from taking a complete break from exercise. Perhaps, listening to an unconscious wisdom, you already have. Then you will be ready to start again from zero. One way to do that is to take a walk in nature, a very slow, short walk. Promise yourself that you will respect your own comfort and not push yourself into a workout. If you are extremely obese, your walk might be only two minutes long. That is fine. Give yourself full permission to do it "as long as I want to and as fast as I want to." As with food, you are practicing self-trust and self-respect.

When you stop imposing exercise upon yourself, then your body's natural desire to move will emerge. You will be called into movement. That is your nature! Think of the words we use to describe someone who is fully alive:

dynamic, active, vibrant. You don't need to coerce yourself into exercise; all you need is to reconnect to your true nature.

Another great way to rediscover the joy and freedom of movement is through dance. All forms of dance are wonderful, but if you are out of practice or just self-conscious, you might need to go back to basics. Find yourself a private space outdoors or in an empty room (without too many things to bump into), and just start moving. Slowly and gently explore all the different ways you can move and hold your body. Especially explore any movements that might seem silly or weird. This is your body and it is your right and freedom to move it any way you want to.

Again, before you do this natural movement activity, give yourself full permission to do it "for as long as I want to." Don't promise yourself that you'll do it for at least ten or twenty minutes. You might find that "as long as I want to" might be longer than you think it is. Usually when we stop doing something we enjoy, it is often because of a semi-conscious anxiety. There's work to be done! You can't afford just to enjoy yourself and do whatever you want, can you? In exploring natural movement or walking, you give yourself permission to go as long or as short as you want to. You allow yourself to do Just This, to put aside all other obligations until you are good and ready. This time is just for you.

In contrast to a workout, where time ticks by so slowly and you force yourself to carry on until the end, can you imagine hardly being able to quit? That is your birthright, the pleasure of movement, and that is what you are reclaiming with this practice.

Will you burn calories this way? Of course you will, but that is just a side-effect. It is not the motivation. If your secret motivation is to burn calories, then you won't be able to give yourself full permission to move as much and as long as you want to. You won't rediscover the joy of movement, and you will always need to motivate yourself or threaten yourself to exercise. And you know the eventual results of that! No, the time for struggle is over.

Another obstacle that thwarts the natural joy of movement is the general alienation from the body that is so common in our culture. We live in a culture of the mind. Higher social status goes to people who work in the mental realm than to people who work with their hands. We are trained from an early age to think rather than feel. If you have a problem, you are supposed to "figure it out". So accustomed are we to thinking rather than feeling, that many of us have almost forgotten how to feel. We accept input from the head rather than the body. Sometimes when I ask someone, "How do you feel about that," they answer, "I think I feel..." Or they say, "I don't know." In my own case, I sometimes notice myself trying to figure out what I should feel, rather than simply and honestly feeling whatever sensations and emotions are really there.

If you cannot feel, then you cannot know what you want or what you like, because the way to know it is to feel it. Knowing does not come through information, it does not come through reason, and it does not come through figuring it out. Knowing comes through feeling. We can read and think and thereby know *about* food and know *about* exercise, but we cannot know food or know exercise that way.

Remember, your body wants to feel good! If you don't know the joy of movement, then you won't want to do it and you'll have to use self-forcing instead. Movement will be a chore, and your exercise session an ordeal from which you try to distract yourself by listening to your headphones or watching the TV in front of the stationary bike.

No wonder so many people say they hate to exercise! Of course they do, because they choose forms of exercise they hate. They choose exercise they hate because they don't know what they like, and they don't know what they like because they do not feel.

If you do not feel, you cannot know what feels good. Not knowing what feels good, you will accept input from your head, your reason, your information sources instead about what is "good for you". Think about that phrase, "good for you". Who is "you"? Whether we are talking about diet or exercise, it assumes that the world is full of millions of identical "you's". But each of us is unique. The only way to know what is good for you, and I mean *you*, is to access knowledge that is as unique as you are. That knowledge comes from your body, your unique vantage point on the world.

The types of workouts that dominate today are a sad statement on life. They contribute to feelings of futility and despair. Treadmills: plodding on and on but getting nowhere. Stationary bikes: exerting an enormous amount of effort to keep a machine running but again, going nowhere yourself. A stair machine: endlessly climbing to the top but never actually getting any higher. A running track: exhausting yourself running around in circles. A swimming pool: back and forth, back and forth in a confined space where you stay in your lane. Weight lifting machines: lifting huge burdens without, in the end, actually moving anything anywhere. From a very simple, commonsense perspective, when you finish a workout you have accomplished essentially nothing. The weights are still sitting there. You haven't gone anywhere. This, I believe, is the deep reason for our impatience with exercising merely to burn calories. The spirit rebels at the unproductive use of life energy.

So how can we reconnect with the body, reconnect with feeling, and thereby tap into the joy of movement that will automatically draw us into an active, dynamic, mobile, and therefore slim body shape? Paradoxically, the first step is often to slow down—slow down and pay attention.

It is the same as with eating. Remember, you can only pay attention to one thing at a time. If your attention is not truly on your food, you will never know in your body what gives you pleasure, and therefore you will never know how to meet your needs (because it is pleasurable to meet your needs). When you exercise, you need to pay attention to what you are doing in order to experience the joy of movement. If you are doing exercise you hate, plodding along on a treadmill or exercise bike, then it is no wonder you want to pay attention to something else. You want to get it over with. If you listen to headphones or watch a television, then your attention is not on your body! More subtly, if you are motivating yourself by thinking of all the calories you are burning and how great you will look, your attention again is not on your body. It is not in the present. If you are watching the clock— only eight minutes left!—and thinking about your next activity (perhaps a large slice of cake to reward yourself for burning all those calories) then again, your attention is not in the present and not in your body.

These kinds of motivational tricks may work for a while, but they are a kind of self-forcing that cannot work in the long run. Your own experience has shown you that. The only sustainable exercise is exercise you enjoy, that you look forward to. Your body naturally desires pleasure, so let's tap into the joy of movement!

The habit of trying to get it over with and trying to pass the time quickly extends beyond exercise. If you have a dull job, you might do the same thing at work. If you don't enjoy school, you might do the same thing with your lessons. Get it over with as painlessly as possible and move on to something you like. Dessert!

The sad thing is that this habit is so powerful it infects activities we enjoy too. Generally speaking, we live constantly in the future. Whenever we try to slow down and enjoy the moment, a relentless anxiety taps us on the shoulder and says, "You can't afford to just do this." Even when you are eating dessert, you might find your attention has moved forward again. "Say, how about *another* dessert after this one?" We can't even keep our attention on the things that give us pleasure! That is why we don't know in our bodies the foods we truly like, and that is why we don't know in our bodies the joy of movement. It is quite ironic, isn't it? The reason you are fat might be because you are not allowing yourself enough pleasure. Society tends to think that fat people are just too indulgent, too greedy, too pleasure-oriented, but it might be the opposite is true.

If you practice the slow walking or movement suggestion above, you will have a chance to hear the voice of anxiety loud and clear. You might find yourself actually enjoying the luxury of moving slowly and taking your time, but a voice will disturb you by saying things like, "This is boring," "I have things to do," "I can't afford to waste this time." When we are doing nothing, we call this voice boredom. Anxiety and boredom are closely related. We are rarely OK with doing nothing at all, so we feel compelled to fill up our empty moments with entertainment or, very often, with eating. The anxiety, the discomfort with doing nothing, prevents us from experiencing the pleasure of doing nothing, which is the pleasure of just being. Similarly, in the realm of exercise, anxiety blocks the pleasure of movement, and in food it blocks the pleasure and fulfillment to be had from simple, natural foods.

This is why doing nothing at all can actually help you lose weight! It is amazing but it is true. If you can allow yourself the pleasure of just being, you are practicing allowing yourself the pleasure of moving and eating. Doing nothing, this zero-calorie activity, will help you lose weight. Unless you have a meditation practice, I bet you have not done this very often, maybe not since you were a child. Most people fill up every empty moment with television, food, or something "productive". There is always something to do. Well, it is time to try something different. It is time to add a little nothing into your life and see what happens.

By far the best place to do nothing is in a natural setting. When you go for a slow walk in nature, empty your mind of any agenda, goal, or expectation. Fill your senses with the natural sight of the wild plants, the sounds of the insects, birds, and wind, the shapes of trees and clouds, the smells of the outdoors, and the sensations of moving your body. You don't have to try to enjoy them. You don't have to constantly evaluate to see whether it is "working". You don't have to justify spending this time.

This is your own sweet time. It is just for you, to have without deserving it and without justifying it. Can you see how giving this gift to yourself will help you feel fed? Can you see how the sights and sounds of nature will fill you with the lost connections so lacking in modern society?

You don't have to *do* anything. The sights, sounds, and smells of nature are healing all by themselves. All you have to "do" is to accept it. No effort is necessary. Can you wrap your mind around that? The age of trying is over. The age of struggle is over. You have tried and tried and tried to be thin, and it hasn't worked. Now you are ready to stop trying and accept your birthright, freely available all the time. Empty yourself and accept.

Even by itself, a frequent treat of time "just for you" in nature can dramatically transform your body and your life. Add to it the Three Mantras of food sanity, and the effect can be downright revolutionary. There is nothing difficult about it. You are not embarking upon some huge, forbidding ordeal. You are letting it be easy.

If you decide to take up another form of joyful movement, such as yoga, dance, or Tai Chi, allow yourself the pleasure of doing nothing but that during the time you do it. Because the habits of anxiety are so deeply ingrained, it is helpful before you start to reassure that scared inner child by saying, "It is OK to do this and only this. Everything else can wait. This is sacred time." Then you will be able to feel the full pleasure of your chosen activity, and that pleasure will draw you back to it again and again.

Traditionally, one way people make themselves do workouts is to punish themselves if they quit. You may have tried this before, punishing yourself with insults like "lazy," "undisciplined" or "weak", creating a whole story about how pathetic you are. Do you really think you can scare yourself into working out? No, actually the eventual effect is the opposite. Human beings are not meant to be slaves. If you apply this kind of self-forcing, sooner or later you will naturally rebel against it. Eventually you will disregard the rewards of self-praise and the punishment of self-criticism. It doesn't work for food, and it won't work for exercise either. You rebel by bingeing or by refusing to exercise even a little bit. This rebellion is one reason why people think they hate exercise, or despair of ever starting an exercise program.

If that is the case, then good for you! This book does not recommend a dietary or exercise "program". No program is needed. However, it might be necessary to unlearn your acquired, rebellious antipathy toward exercise. Letting go of the calorie-burning mentality is a good start. It is also helpful to give yourself full permission to stop any time. Tell yourself that you can stop after ten minutes, after five minutes, even after one minute if you don't want to carry on. And, promise yourself that you will not punish yourself when you stop. You will not be disappointed in yourself that you only exercised for five minutes. By stopping when you truly want to stop, you deprogram the exercise=self-forcing equation and short-circuit the resistance and rebelliousness. You nurture self-trust.

"I can stop whenever I want" actually has two meanings. The first meaning is obvious; the second meaning is, "I don't have to stop until I really want to." You give your unconscious mind permission to enact its true desires. And remember, true desires come from true needs, and when you fulfill true needs, the craving for substitutes goes away.

With this full permission to move for as long as you want, and as slowly as you want, you might find yourself spending more and more time in movement. You might go for hours without stopping, you might naturally start running from a walk, or doing more strenuous yoga. That's fine, but make sure not to become attached to this outcome. Don't set it as a goal, and if it happens, don't set it as your new standard. Always keep your permission to self fresh and real. Your body will go through various phases as it recovers vibrant, active health. There may be times when it is most appropriate to rest and rebuild. If you have been doing hourslong walks every day, and all of a sudden you wake up one morning and it seems a chore, then don't force yourself.

Remember, the goal and the method of this book is to reconnect with the pleasure of being alive. Movement is one of those pleasures. Even if you aren't burning many calories, the joy of movement will help bring you more fully to life. To be alive is to feel. Feel fully the pleasure of moving your body, and you will naturally come more and more alive. To be fully alive is to be healthy, vibrant and fit. These are the results of fully feeling.

Chapter Eighteen

Meeting the Need

Once upon a time there was a man who lost his house key. There he was, pacing up and down under the streetlight, looking for his key. A passerby approached and said, "Sir, you seem to have lost something, can I help you find it?"

"Yes, alas," said the man, "I have lost my house key."

"Okay, I'll help you look," said the passerby. "Now tell me, where were you when you dropped it?"

"I think it was when I was getting something out of my pocket, over there near those trees."

"Over there by the trees! Tell me then, if you lost it over there, why are you looking for it over here?"

The man explained, "It is much too dark over there. I am looking here under the streetlight, where I can see!"

Many of us are in the same situation as that man. We have lost something very important—the key to our homecoming, the key to our birthright of vitality and health. But rather than venture into the shadows, the dark unknown, the places we are afraid to go, we search and search for the solution in the same old, familiar area. For the obese person, that safe, familiar area could be the realm of food. She searches and searches that realm, trying out all kinds of diets, all kinds of motivational techniques, all kinds of supplements, programs, and plans.

Nothing works. That is because for her, the key is not to be found in the area of food. I have already explained why: food is only a substitute for another need. What is that need? It is different for every person, but it probably lies in the shadows. It is somewhere you are afraid to go. Very likely, you know exactly what it is! You are just afraid to venture there and pick up that key.

If you are eating to comfort and distract yourself from an unfulfilling relationship or a career you don't believe in, you know exactly what I am talking about.

I would like to give you a small exercise you can do to help bring greater awareness to the deep and hidden needs that generate binges and food addictions. Remember, desires come from unmet needs. That also means that desires offer a clue, a portal to those needs. If you practice the Three Mantras of food sanity, these deep unmet needs will begin to become more apparent already. The following exercise is designed to meet them directly.

Keep in mind as you do this that you are not required to DO anything about the unmet need. We are releasing all self-forcing. The fear of "having to do something about it" might prevent you from even going there. It is what keeps the unmet need in the dark. This exercise is merely to bring it to light. That does not mean you won't do anything about it. It's just that when you do, the action will feel natural and right.

Step 1: Let's start with what's on the surface: with desire. Divide a piece of paper into two columns and make a list of all the things you want. Don't be shy! Feel free to list your most superficial, frivolous desires, even your nasty ones. Remember, this isn't a plan for action, this is just a realistic inventory of where you are right now. Here are some examples to get you started:

"I want an iPod."

"I want lots of money."

"I want to be treated like a queen."

"I want a really hot girlfriend."

"I want my children to call more often."

"I want to spend quality time with my grandchildren."

"I want to smash something."

"I want a box of cookies right now."

"I want to eat all the food in the house."

"I want people to like me."

"I want to be thin."

"I want to be beautiful."

"I want my spouse to be more considerate."

"I want a new car."

"I want straight A's."

"I want my son to get straight A's."

"I want my daughter to break up with that biker."

"I want to be popular."

"I want to be normal."

"I want to feel good."

"I want to die."

"I want my health problem to disappear."

"I want so-and-so to get what's coming to him."

"I want so-and-so to apologize."

"I want to feel safe."

"I want people to listen to me."

"I want to know if there is a God."

Step 2: In the second column, write down the deeper desire underneath each of the desires in the first column. For example, if you want a lot of money, think about why you want that. What would it bring you? Maybe what you really want is to feel secure in the world, or to feel free, or to be respected. You might even take it yet another level deeper. Why do you want to be respected? Why do you crave security, when someday you will die anyway? What is it you really want?

If you get stuck on any of these, a good way to find the underlying need or desire is to imagine yourself actually achieving the desire in the first column. Imagine the feeling of obtaining the object of your desire. And then imagine how you would feel after the thrill or feeling of gratification has worn off. If it is a substitute for something deeper, then you will still have a wanting underneath, a longing. What is it you want now? Many Olympic athletes, a few days or weeks or months after winning the gold medal, have a huge sense of letdown, of emptiness. They have achieved what they thought was their greatest desire, but it wasn't enough. The longing, the hunger is still there. It is exactly the same as the feeling of being stuffed with food and still being hungry.

When people work through the surface desires to get to the deep ones, the same few items come up again and again. To love and to be loved. To know. To be known. To explore. To learn. To create. To play. To experience pleasure. To enjoy beauty. Whether in a prison or a country club, all human beings have the same fundamental desires. Ultimately, they underlie everything we strive for. Even the most greedy and violent desires are rooted in these beautiful, divine qualities. Greed and violence are what happen when our divine basic desires are denied and twisted and diverted toward substitutes.

I know that if you look within, you can sense the basic goodness of your true being. This is the basic goodness we are accessing and learning to trust in Transformational Weight Loss. Because goodness is our true nature, we don't have to struggle and fight to attain it. That includes goodness in the form of a beautiful, healthy body.

When you have gone through your list of true desires, spend a few moments appreciating your basic goodness. It can be very moving to look at a greedy or violent desire, and realize, "All I really wanted was to express love. All I really wanted was to like myself."

Step 3: As you went through your list, there was probably one need or desire that stood out for you, something that you recognize as the Big Issue in your life right now. It might be associated with a whole scenario of a relationship, money, career, or health. Identify this most prominent desire, including all of its more superficial expressions. Then spend a few minutes with it, just feeling it. Feel what it is like to *want*. Feel what it is like to have this unmet need. Remember, you don't have to do anything about it right now. Most of all, you don't have to "figure out" what you are going to do. You don't need to find an answer. You don't need to find a way out. Don't go down that road. That is the road of trying hard, of struggle, and ultimately of despair. It is enough just to be there, to be and to feel.

I call this exercise "Meeting the Need," not because it immediately fulfills the need, but in the sense of "Hello, pleased to meet you." You meet the need, you become acquainted with it. You have ventured into the shadows where the key is. The next step will be to use the key, and you will know exactly when and how to do that when the time comes. In fact, by simply putting your full loving attention on the true desire, you set an unstoppable chain of events in motion. You might not see the results for a while, or you might see them very soon. You will act when the time is right. You won't be able to stop yourself.

Chapter Nineteen

Food for the Spirit

Not just the substances you put into your mouth, but anything you bring into your being is a kind of food. Some examples are breath, sights, sounds, sensations, ideas, stories, and beliefs. The way you bring something into your being is simply to pay attention to it. Then it enters your world and becomes part of your self.

That is why, if you eat while watching TV, you won't feel very fed by that food. Your attention is mostly on the television program, not on what you are eating. You are feeding yourself television! In the same way, if you eat while obsessing about calories, whether it is "good for you", thoughts of "just one more after this", thoughts of dessert, and so on, then what you are actually eating is thoughts, worries, and obsessions. No wonder you keep eating and eating. Your body hardly knows it has had food.

It is written, "Man cannot live by bread alone." In order to be nourished (and not use ordinary food as a substitute), we need to fill ourselves with nourishing sensations, thoughts, and experiences as well. The second mantra of food sanity was, "I give myself full permission to eat whatever I want." Well, why not extend that to other kinds of food too? When the urge to "have something" arises, pause for a moment to ask yourself what it is you really want. Maybe it is not food;

maybe you habitually substitute food for something else, and maybe that something else is obvious.

The substitute desire is not always hidden. We eat when we are tired, we eat when we are lonely, we eat when we are bored. Sometimes, if you pause for just a moment, the true need will become apparent.

If the true need is not apparent, maybe that is because it has gone unmet for so long that you are numb to the hunger that it generates. To restore sensitivity to true needs, you can do the same thing I suggested for food: add more kinds of "real food" to the menu. In other words, explore some of the other "foods" listed above.

For example, suppose the desire to have something arises, and you pause for a moment and realize that you are not actually hungry for food, but you don't know what you want. So, try some things. Have a few sips of water—maybe you were actually thirsty. Some experts claim that most Americans are chronically dehydrated, having ignored the sensation of thirst for so long that they no longer recognize it.

If it is not thirst, then try something else. The empty feeling could well be a sign of "nature deficit disorder". The human nervous system is designed to be filled all day with the sights, sounds, and smells of nature. If you take a few minutes to listen intently to the birds singing, you will feel enriched, filled with a connection that food used to serve. For this to work, you have to really listen to the songs, not just treat them as background noise. You have to put your attention on them and bring them into your being. You can do the same with the other senses. Spend a few minutes filling your vision with the sight of a tree or flower. Just empty your mind and allow the plant to fill you. I cannot explain it in any other way, because it is something you already know how to do. Don't try to figure out why or whether or how, just go out and do it! Or go out barefoot and fill your being with the sensation of grass under your feet.

Often, people use food as a substitute for attention, a pattern which you might trace back to childhood. In a sense, food *is* a way to pay attention to yourself, but it is often not the kind of attention you need, especially when uncomfortable emotions come up. This is somewhat ironic, because like other kinds of pain, these emotions are nothing other than a call for attention. Their purpose is to call attention to an unmet need. So, if you feel that old familiar craving, that wanting, coming up, try just giving it a little attention. Witness it, feel it, give it space inside you. That might just be the attention you need instead of food. Even if you don't feel any strong emotions, give yourself attention sometimes anyway, a few sweet moments just for you. We all need attention. You've probably noticed how children go to great lengths to obtain it from adults. We are no different, really, except that we are the adult.

Here is an essential point: none of these activities are tricks to take your mind off food or to delay your next eating binge. They are not new ways of controlling or denying yourself. After all, it could be that your hunger really is for food. The attitude to adopt when you bring water, birds, or plants into your being is an attitude of pleasure and indulgence. You are opening yourself to the deliciousness of life itself. It feels good to meet your needs. That is a truth that will never change. It feels good to meet your needs, and you are exploring more and more ways to do that. Then you will no longer try to fill all those needs with food.

At bottom, food is just one of the ways we connect with a nourishing universe. Therefore, anything we do to strengthen our connections to the rest of humanity and the rest of life will diminish the desire for food. Planting a garden, which connects you to the soil, insects, flowers, and weeds in a very concrete, sensual way, is therefore a great way to lose weight that has nothing to do with the calories expended. The same goes for taking care of pets or children— really giving them love and attention, not just trying to get through the day. This is important. Often women put on weight when they have young children. Food becomes in this case a substitute, an escape from the loneliness, boredom, and stress of suburban mothering.

The loneliness, ill health, disconnection, and obesity of modern life all go together. They are the automatic free side dishes of a car-based, television-based, computer-based, money-based, modern lifestyle. They are part of an overall pattern, a pattern that hurts. The things we do to alleviate the discomfort often intensify the pattern: watching TV to assuage loneliness, eating snack foods to alleviate boredom and sweets to feel a moment of intimacy. When you change one part of this pattern, for example returning to real food, you will be irresistibly drawn toward authenticity in other aspects of life too. You will seek out real nourishment for the spirit. As with food, real nourishment is readily available. Usually it is only habit and ignorance that prevents us from accessing it. We live in a fundamentally abundant, all-providing universe.

Because anything we bring into our being is food, you can apply the principles of this book to any choice in life. Choose with full license, and commit to feeling fully the results of your choices. Then you will come into alignment with

your natural desires, and discover the effortless goodness of
your true being.

Chapter Twenty

In the Absence of Hope

Sometimes you might find yourself face to face with a need you believe you cannot possibly meet. You might be quite clear that you need to be in nature, but all you can afford is an apartment next to the interstate highway. You might know your need for creative self-expression, but be stuck in a dull dead-end job. You may be quite clear that you need human intimacy, but who would want to be with fat, ugly, divorced you? So of course you eat and eat and eat.

Overeating is one way people respond when they feel victimized by life. I would like to clear up some confusion about victim mentality that you find even in spiritual writings. Like fear, victim mentality is not an enemy to fight against. It is merely a symptom that points to unmet needs. On the one hand, what the spiritual books say is true: you are the creator of your life and in no sense its victim. On the other hand, the economic, social, and political forces that oppress and impoverish people are real as well. Moreover, victim mentality harbors yet another aspect of truth: there is no rational, practical way out of your predicament.

Have you ever had those annoying conversations where a well-meaning friend starts giving you practical suggestions? "Have you tried eating less?" "How about joining a gym?" "Have you sent out your résumé?" "You could hire a publicist!" "Have you tried to reason with him?" "You just need to organize your time better." And to each suggestion, you come up with a rebuttal—why it wouldn't work. Both people leave the conversation feeling frustrated. The helpful friend feels frustrated because you obviously won't accept help, you refuse to take action, and you are wallowing in your victimhood. You feel frustrated too, because your friend just doesn't get it, can't put herself in your shoes, doesn't understand your situation. You might feel vaguely insulted as well, because someone else is assuming that it is so easy—if only you would do this and do that. The implication is that you simply are weak, lazy, lacking in motivation or self-discipline. But the truth is that you are not going to get out of your condition by trying harder.

Fortunately, you don't have to. The exit from the condition of the victim is not through trying harder. As with obesity, its frequent partner, the way out is to meet the true need. So what is the need that victim mentality signals? There are at least two needs here. One is the need for whatever the victim story uses as its fodder: money, connection, and so on. But these needs can exist apart from victim mentality, and I have explained how to "meet" them in the section, "Meeting the Need".

Victim mentality arises from a story we build around an unmet need or wound. One would think that we are "wallowing" in that wound, but the opposite is true. The story is an escape from feeling it. Instead of feeling the pain from the wound itself, we put our attention on the emotions associated with the story. These emotions are a substitute for what we really want, which is to feel and to heal the unmet need at the core. Like any substitute, they are addictive. To maintain the addiction, we unconsciously perpetuate the circumstances that include the woundedness. We perpetuate the loneliness, the poverty, or the obesity.

Victim mentality is related to overeating in another way too. We use it to feel deserving, to obtain permission to be good to ourselves, and to comfort ourselves. Food becomes its vehicle, but of course then we are not eating out of hunger.

Victim mentality arises out of neediness, and perpetuates the neediness. To exit it, shift your focus from the victim story onto the need itself. Feel what it is like to be lonely. Feel what it is like to be bored. Feel what it is like to be anxious and afraid for your future. Be sure to focus on the feeling itself and not the story. Feel the anxiety, and not the story of "I don't have enough money to pay the rent next week, and so I'm going to see an eviction notice on my door, and the police will come, and the collection agency is going to take further action, and they're going to shut off the electricity..." All of these things might come to pass, but right now you are going to focus on the feeling, not the story. The feeling is of panic or anxiety. Feel it! And keep feeling it until it passes. It won't last long if you don't maintain the story around it.

Please understand that by doing this, you are not abandoning taking action on any of your practical problems. When you have fully felt the need, action will be natural, clear and decisive. You will know exactly what to do when the time comes.

So you see, victim mentality is really just a call for attention. We use it sometimes to get attention from others, but the real source of the attention you need is you! It is a call to pay attention to yourself—not your stories, your *self*. That is the real need. Be with yourself, be with yourself, be with yourself, in solitude, in nature, and throughout all your activities of the day. Do not seek to justify this need to yourself or others, and please do not broadcast it. Keep it a secret. This self-intimacy is sacred, it is just for you.

Soon you will not want to be a victim any more. You won't have conquered victim mentality—you will have outgrown it. You will shed it as a snake sheds its skin. Familiar with the true needs, you will access the power to meet those needs. You will reach for what you want. You will feel free to do this, because you will have fallen in love with yourself. And, because you will realize that your self is of identical essence with all those other selves out there, you will fall in love with the world too.

Chapter Twenty-one

Because I want to

One of the best things I have ever done for my body and my life was to stop justifying everything I do. To need to justify everything is slavery. You might be familiar with that mentality in your eating, justifying everything according to how many calories or fat or carbs it has, or if it is "good for you", or what else you ate that day or did that day to deserve it.

The goal of this book is to eventually replace all those justifications with a single, new justification—or actually, a non-justification. The only reason you need to do anything is, "Because I want to." That is where the Three Mantras of Food Sanity will take you. Because your sensitivity to your true wants will grow as you devote attention to the feelings associated with food, "because I want to" will evolve over time. Soon you will no longer say, "I'm not having ice cream because it is bad for me and has 380 calories." You will say, "I'm not having any, because I just don't want to."

Or, as the case may be, you will no longer say, "I am going to have some ice cream because I ate a small dinner and worked out today and besides, I'm feeling sad and I need some." You will say, "I am going to have some ice cream, because I want to."

As with food, so with life. That feeling of "I hardly dare believe it is true" can extend to give license to live your true desires. As with food, nothing bad is going to happen to you when you cease the effort of control. You will be cast into a new world, and that can be scary. Remember the fallacy inherent in the word "selfish"—it implies that the self is bad. Is life a struggle or isn't it? You decide. I, for one, am tired of the struggle. And so I gave it up, and life changed in ways I could hardly have imagined.

Unconsciously, I had been living in a slave relationship to my spouse, to my work, and to all the people around me. Always seeking to please others, I didn't even know what my true desires were. If asked, "What restaurant do you want to go to?" I would immediately try to figure out what would please the other. I did not realize that people have a real desire to please me, just as much as I desire to please them. One of life's greatest pleasures is to please another person, and it is a generous gift to allow another the opportunity to please you. But I had been in a different kind of pattern. One day I decided I was going to live for myself. I remember it was a small thing. I changed my mind about a trip, and I was asked to justify myself. "Why are you changing your mind? I was expecting you to go. You said that. You can't change your mind without a good reason." But I had no reason to offer except, "Because I want to." I could hardly bear to say those words for my fear, but I think that was the most liberating sentence I ever spoke.

We are beings of desire. Desire is the essence of life, and to suppress desire is to be half-alive. Desire will guide us toward goodness, it will guide us toward life, it will guide us toward health. But only true desire will do this, not the substitutes for what we really want. That is why it is important to feel everything, because by feeling we know pleasure, and by knowing pleasure we know what we want because it feels good to meet our needs!

You can be free. A free person does what she wants. "What about responsibility?" you might ask. Just like everything else that is healthy or good, we see responsibility as yet another struggle against desire. That too is an illusion. It can be a pleasure to meet your responsibilities. Those that it is not a pleasure to meet, well, you might begin to question whether they truly serve your interests or the interests of people around you. Have you ever oh-so-irresponsibly quit a job, or started showing up late and gotten fired, only to find a new occupation that never would have appeared had you been at the old job?

It may also be that the same confusion that affects food also affects other areas of life, so that you don't really know what gives you pleasure. I find it pleasurable to serve the needs of my children, even to clean up my 2-year-old's "accidents". I find it pleasurable to make good food for them and to wash the dishes. You can access this pleasure by focusing your attention on the real purpose of what you are doing, the real motivation. You can even choose which of your many complex motivations you will focus on, and begin to see everything you do as a gift. Try it, it feels really good!

In his book *Nonviolent Communication*, Marshall Rosenberg offers a great way to access the real purpose of the things we think we "have to" do. He suggests replacing all "have to" sentences with "I choose to... because...." The unconscious habit of saying "I have to" is central in stripping us of our sovereignty over our lives. When I first became aware of this habit, I was amazed at how many times an hour or a minute I would say "I have to." Now I follow Rosenberg's advice. If I catch myself saying, "I have to go home and make dinner now," I rephrase it as, "I choose to go home and make dinner now, because it is my joy to feed my children healthy food prepared with love." Other times, I may discover that the "have to" doesn't have a solid foundation in my joy or desire. When you replace, "I have to stay married" with "I choose to stay married because I am afraid of people judging me," then you might be moved to make a different choice. There is no more fooling yourself that you have to.

I would like you to remove all "have to's" and "should's" from your vocabulary. Have-to's and should's are agents of victim mentality that deny freedom by their very meaning. You can replace them with other ways of thinking that affirm your sovereignty over your life. For example, Louise Hay gives a useful exercise of replacing "should" sentences with, "If I really wanted to, I could..." This rephrasing taps into very different beliefs about the world. The power over your life returns to you.

You can apply variations of both these replacements to your relationship with food. When you eat something, affirm your autonomy by saying, "I choose to eat this, because..." Be honest. It could be "because I'm hungry", "because I'm depressed," "because I want to be polite" "because I'm bored" "because it is dinner time." You don't need to take any further action. Simply being in the truth will have an effect.

Similarly, instead of saying, "I should eat less sugar" you can say, "If I really wanted to, I could eat less sugar." "If I really wanted to, I could exercise." Then you come face to face with the possibility that you just don't want to right now. At the same time, you affirm your ability and license to fulfill your desires. Because if you want to, you can. You are permitted. Why? Just because you want to.

Chapter Twenty-two

The Power to Choose

In *The Yoga of Eating* I wrote that there is a proper role for self-discipline and willpower. It is not to control yourself. It is to bring the wisdom you discover in moments of clarity and attention to those other moments of your life when you do not feel clear. In times of connection to true desire and true pleasure, you can make a structure for yourself to extend that knowledge into the rest of your life.

For example, say you drink a cup of coffee and pay attention to the effects in your body, and have a clear, strong realization that you don't feel good at all. You might make a rule for yourself of "I don't drink coffee." Then when someone offers you a cup at the office, you can say no even if, at that moment, you are too preoccupied to let the answer come from your body.

The recovery of authentic desire usually takes some time. In my life, it took a long time for me to undo the habits of self-forcing and get in touch with what I really wanted. There may be times when you truly don't know if you want a cookie right now. At those times, you can fall back upon the rules and structure you created for yourself at the time you did know.

The structure you create for yourself might be very strict and detailed. Just be sure to reconnect it frequently to the authentic knowing that comes from fully experiencing food. Your needs change over time, and you don't want to be stuck in a dogmatic system that was right for you last year but not today. Always be honest with yourself. Is this structure working? How you will know is very simple. Just pay attention to how it makes you feel. You should feel great! If your structure becomes a chore, an apparatus of self-denial, then it is high time you reconnected to pleasure and desire.

As you develop the Three Mantras of Food Sanity and apply them more and more consistently, you will have less and less need for rules and structures. You will know what you want, you will want what makes you feel good, and what feels good will make you healthy. There will be no rules and no self-denial. Want and need will be perfectly aligned.

In the five years since I wrote *The Yoga of Eating*, I have discovered another dimension of self-discipline more fundamental than what I have just described. The first served me well for a long time, which is why I offer it to you. Now I would like to offer you the deeper level. It is based on the realization that our only true power is to choose what we pay attention to. True self-discipline, then, is to stay in the realization of that power.

Remember, whatever we pay attention to is our food. Whatever we pay attention to, we bring into ourselves and with it, create our being. From that being, all other decisions flow automatically. We think we are choosing them, but we are not. The real choice happened long before, when we created ourselves as the being that would make such a decision. In other words, you are out of control! The only thing you can actually control is your attention. Everything else flows from that.

When you finally stop bingeing and overeating, it won't be because you will have brought them under control. That is impossible. It will be because you have paid attention to the experience of doing that, as well as to the pleasure of eating a different way. It will be because you have shifted your attention to your desire and pleasure. That shift in attention will cause a revolution to happen without even trying.

Let your new discipline, then, be to become a master of attention. Cultivate a new habit of choosing consciously what you will pay attention to, and therefore who you will create yourself as. This discipline underlies everything else in this book. When you are a conscious chooser, you can choose to pay attention to the discomfort of overeating, rather than to the thought-form, "I will never do this again." You can choose to pay attention to actual pleasure, rather than whether it is good for you or what you will get from it. You can pay attention to the spiritually nourishing sounds of nature, rather than the constant inner monologue of anxieties. Some things call your attention more loudly than others, and we have habits of where we put our attention, but the choice is always there. Let your discipline be to exercise this choice more and more.

When you do that, your eating habits will change. It will appear that you have become more disciplined in your eating, but that is an illusion. The discipline will be in your attention, which allows you to integrate pleasure and discomfort and to know food in your body. From that will flow a revolution in what you eat and how you eat.

Chapter Twenty-three

Your Body, Your Self

Your body is not an isolated aspect of who you are, and it will not change in isolation either. Obesity is just one facet of a way of thinking, a way of eating, a way of seeing yourself, a way of presenting yourself. It is part of how you know yourself, your stories about the past, your expectations for the future, and your beliefs about the world. It is *who you have been* for a long time.

You are about to leave behind much that is familiar. Are you ready for everything I just listed to change? Most diet books tell you to eat different things; this book asks you to eat in a different way. Then, naturally, you will find yourself eating different things. It will be a part of who you are becoming. For your weight to change, much else must change along with it. Does that seem like a tall order? After all, you couldn't even change your diet, and now I'm saying you are going to have to change much more than that? Be at peace. The change does not require your struggle, but only your cooperation. You are being born into a new self, propelled by the contracting womb of your circumstances. There is no more room for you there, in the self-world you once inhabited.

I am not saying you will take no action. To cooperate with the birthing is to act in accordance with its rhythms. It is your desires that will do the pushing. I think you can feel it now. It is the desire to get real. This book is about getting real with food and getting real with yourself. Because your real self is vibrant, vital, and vigorous, not sick and fat. I have offered you many ways of getting real: real food, real sensations, natural sounds. Back to the body. Meeting real needs. Doubtless you will be attracted to other ways of being real too, that I haven't described in this book. For example, you might notice a desire to get real in your communication by refraining from gossip, lies, and talking behind people's backs. And this won't be a discipline, it will be a *desire*, because it feels so good to be pure of word. You might also want to get real in your listening, by focusing on the other person and not on your own stream of silent judgments. You might desire as well to get real in your work, and find ways of creatively expressing your gifts toward a purpose you really care about. Finally, your growing desire to be real might give you new courage to act from your true nature of love, so that in each situation the old unconscious habit of "What can I get from this" gives way to the new and pleasurable thought-pattern, "What can I give?"

All of this, and much more, is what you are moving toward. This book is just one step along the way. Other books and teachers are coming to you soon!

Your years of patient struggle were not wasted. You developed strength, patience, endurance, and a capacity for joy in the midst of hardship and despair that is going to empower your gifts in the new state of life that awaits you. Nothing was in vain, and there are no mistakes. You are going to have a distinct advantage over people who were never obese: the miracle that is happening in your body will give you a sense of expanded possibilities. Yes, miracles can happen! You are about to experience one. The process has started already, and it will unfold as naturally and inevitably as a flower unfolds from the bud or a butterfly from a cocoon. Losing weight is only one aspect it, your gateway to the rest. Now it is time to step fully into your process of metamorphosis, with eagerness, serenity, and faith.

Printed in the United States
215259BV00001B/57/A

9 780977 622214